DATE DUE		
MAR 2 6 1991			
MAY 1 4 1991			
5-24-91			

Biography & Autobiography/
Medical

362
TRU

On with my life

ON WITH MY LIFE

ON WITH MY LIFE

PATTI TRULL

G.P. PUTNAM'S SONS, NEW YORK

ACKNOWLEDGMENTS

I would like to thank Vicki Carney for all her help with
ON WITH MY LIFE, and thank her patient family,
Jack, Anna and Erica, as well.

A special thanks goes to my parents, Betty and Jim, and to
Wayne, Cheryl, Annette and Teresa, for all their love and
support through the years.

Library of Congress Cataloging in Publication Data
Trull, Patti.
On with my life.
Summary: Diagnosed as having osteosarcoma at the
age of fifteen and having her leg amputated as a result,
the author relates her determination to overcome a
potentially lethal disease and her later experiences
as a therapist to cancer patients in a children's
hospital.
1. Osteosarcoma—Patients—Washington (State)—
Biography—Juvenile literature. 2. Tumors in children
—Patients—Washington (State)—Biography—Juvenile
literature. 3. Trull, Patti. [1. Trull, Patti.
2. Sick. 3. Osteosarcoma. 4. Cancer. 5. Rehabilita-
tion] I. Title.
RC280.B6T8   1983   362.1'9699471   83-3058
ISBN 0-399-20977-8

*This book is about childhood cancer. It is not, however,
about death and dying—it is about life and living, and courage.
To the children who are no longer here, it is written as a legacy
of love; to those who are, a legacy of hope.*

The child's philosophy is the true one. He does not despise the bubble because it burst; and he immediately sets to work to blow another.

—*J. J. Procter*

ON WITH MY LIFE

ONE

"HAPPY BIRTHDAY TO YOU . . . HAPPY BIRTHDAY TO you . . . happy birthday, dear Patti . . ." Fifteen years old! I couldn't believe it, only six more months until I could get my driver's permit. I felt great that day; Mom had made dinner and my favorite chocolate cake. My girl friends had come for a slumber party—a night of talking about boys, clothes, sex, hair, parents (mostly mothers), and all the other things that eight fifteen-year-olds can talk about until three in the morning.

It was September and we had just started high school. It was exciting, but getting used to a larger school, new teachers, changing classes, and making new friends meant a big adjustment for all of us. We were struggling to find out who we were and where we fit in. School had suddenly become serious stuff with people talking about grades and college. I personally couldn't imagine anyone wanting to go to school if they didn't have to, and worse yet, paying for it. I was definitely not interested in college or grades—I just wanted to get through high school and have a good time at football games, drill team, Pep Club, driving, and being with friends.

I baby-sat and did housekeeping for a family down the

street. They had two children whom I enjoyed watching, and I liked the extra money My schedule was busy with three days of baby-sitting, two days of teaching dancing, and drill-team practice and Pep Club squeezed in between. I was exhausted every night but content.

I loved to dance and had taken tap and ballet lessons since I was eight years old. My two younger sisters took dancing, the neighbors took dancing, everyone took dancing! As we grew up, we would go to each other's dance recitals, laugh a lot, sweat a lot, and wonder if any of us would ever go to New York and become famous. I wanted to teach and that's what I did. I helped my instructor with the younger children two days a week and took one lesson a week myself.

I tried other things too. I was a majorette in parades; I played the clarinet for seven days until I decided there was something drastically wrong with my lips; I played the organ for three months, until my teacher got tired of my writing the notes on the keys with a felt-tipped pen because I couldn't read music; I had French lessons for two months before I decided I wasn't ever going to Paris anyway. If I wasn't good at it, I didn't stick with it—my patience was short and I liked instant results.

My right knee began hurting about a month after my birthday. I was all geared up for a girl friend's birthday slumber party but that night I felt more and more uncomfortable. I had a hard time listening to the stereo and couldn't even enjoy the pizza. My leg kept throbbing. I took some aspirin, but it didn't help. I walked around and that didn't help. My knee was hurting, but I couldn't figure out where the pain had come from—or why. I hadn't done anything unusual, just dancing and running track in physical education. Maybe I had pulled a muscle. The pain lasted all night and into the morning. By the time my dad came to pick me up I was close to tears. Why wouldn't it go away? When I got home I took some more aspirin, put a heating pad on my knee, and went to sleep. When I woke up the pain was gone. It didn't come back for three weeks.

I had always been a healthy person with nothing more than a cold or sore throat now and then. I had had a routine physical for high school and was in good health. My teeth were rotting but my body was fine. The dentist had found fifteen cavities and I had been to see him only six months before. That was the end of soft drinks for me. I had never been in the hospital or had any serious illness. I was fine . . . just fine.

As it got closer to Thanksgiving, I was looking forward to skiing. The leaves had fallen. Halloween had come and gone. And I was spending lots of time doing homework, which I hated. Mom had begun to act strangely during those weeks. I couldn't put my finger on it, but she wasn't her usual easy-going self. My parents had been under a lot of stress because both my grandmothers had had strokes within a week of each other and were not expected to live. My mom's mother was in Australia and my other grandmother was in North Carolina so there wasn't much my parents could do since we lived in Seattle, Washington.

On a rainy Sunday afternoon in mid-November I went to Mass and a matinee with my brother, Wayne, and my sisters, Cheryl and Annette. When we got home our parents were unusually serious. I thought that one of my grandmothers had died. Instead, we heard an announcement that was going to change our lives. My mother was pregnant. I couldn't believe it. How could she be pregnant? The baby was not unwanted, but definitely unplanned. Cheryl said she'd rather have a new puppy. Annette thought it was grand. Wayne didn't have an opinion. I was embarrassed. What would the kids at school say?

After a while we started getting used to the idea and became excited. But my mother was exhausted thinking about starting over with diapers and the PTA at forty-two.

And she knew the dangers of having a baby at her age. More than anything, she worried about it being healthy. This next year, 1968, was going to be a big year for changes at the Trull household.

Thanksgiving was lovely. We had our first snow of the year, and I was getting excited about skiing. I was hoping my knee would start feeling better so it wouldn't bother me during conditioning. I had been experiencing a strange pain for a couple of weeks. It would come and go with no predictable pattern. My knee would be fine for days and I would forget about it. Then it would hurt a lot and I would make a doctor's appointment, but before I could keep the appointment, the pain would go away again.

I finally did go and have my knee examined. The X-rays showed nothing wrong. There was no swelling or other abnormality. The doctor suggested that I limit my activity and use an Ace bandage for support.

But it became harder and harder to walk around. The halls at school seemed longer and I was losing my stamina. I was still dancing and trying to run track, but both became more a chore than pleasure.

We gave a dance recital at a local nursing home the first week of December. My leg throbbed before I danced. This was strange because it usually hurt after dancing, not before. I performed better than I ever had but limped back into the dressing room. A sweet old lady asked if I'd rubbed a blister. I thought to myself, I think I've done more than rub a blister. I was in excruciating pain and could hardly walk to the car. That was the last time I ever tap-danced.

I didn't want to tell anyone, but I knew I needed to see a doctor. Oh, how I disliked doctors—no, I hated them. I had never had a bad experience with a doctor, but to me, they meant pain, agony, and needles—not health and healing. I usually had to be bribed with a new dress or lunch out to get me to a doctor's appointment, but this time I didn't care. I just knew that I hurt like hell and something was wrong.

We made an appointment with a new doctor, Dr. Flashman, for the next day. He was an orthopedic surgeon, and although I didn't know what orthopedic meant, I did know what surgeon meant. I was restless and, for some reason, concerned about missing school.

Dr. Flashman's office was large, and a lot of people were in the waiting room. The receptionist was friendly and asked us to fill out the usual new patient and insurance forms. I was nervous about being there, and the smell of alcohol didn't help. What was this doctor going to do? I remembered all the free advice my friends had given me on the phone the night before: "You probably have arthritis," "I'll bet it's just a pulled tendon," "cartilage damage," "he'll probably stick a needle in your knee and poke around to take fluid." Shit! I was trying to concentrate on a magazine when I heard, "Patricia Trull."

This is it, I thought. I just wanted to get it over with, go home, and feel better. The worst that could happen would be I'd have to limit my activities for a while. I got up on the examining table, took off my jeans, and tried to talk to Mom who sat over by the window. We talked about trivial things like what to have for dinner and good names for babies. It was late afternoon and was raining again like it does in Seattle 300 days out of the year. Where was this Dr. Flashman? He was already an hour late!

When he did arive, he began asking a lot of questions.

"Patricia, how long has your knee been hurting?"

"Two months," I answered

"Does it hurt at any certain time of the day or night?"

"More at night."

"Have you noticed any swelling?"

"No."

More questions and more answers. He seemed like a nice man who knew what he was doing. I began to relax as he moved my leg through various positions. He explained that he wanted to get some X-rays. I was cooperative because I knew they were painless. The X-ray technician was just a few years older than I was. She was pleasant and chatted the whole time she was X-raying my right leg from hip to toes. Then I went back to the examining room.

Mom and I waited and talked about Christmas coming, how glad I was she was going to have a baby, and how much fun it would be to start playing Santa Claus again. I wanted a ten-speed bicycle for Christmas and Mom wanted her four children to quit fighting so much. An hour passed before the doctor returned again. He wanted more X-rays. The technician didn't say much this time. It was dark outside and only a few people were still in the office. Our appointment had been at 3:00 and it was close to 6:00 now. My stomach began to hurt and my head ached.

Dr. Flashman finally got back to us and sat down.

"Patricia, we have a problem." (I liked the "we," not "you.") "There appears to be a tumor in your right leg."

He showed me where it was located, in the top part of my right leg in a bone called the femur. He explained that because the other doctor had only x-rayed my knee where the pain was, the tumor had gone undetected. I had experienced what is called "referred pain." The cause of the pain was in the bone that went from my hip to my knee.

The word tumor meant nothing to me. I hadn't known anyone with a tumor, and the diagnosis certainly wasn't what I'd expected to hear. Dr. Flashman told us that he had made arrangements for us to go to Children's Hospital the following day for more tests and X-rays. The word "hospital" scared me and I began to cry.

"I can't go to the hospital. People who are really sick go to hospitals. I only have something wrong with my leg."

Mom was crying too, but not because of the word "hospital"—she had heard the word "tumor." Dr. Flashman told us to go home, get a good night's sleep and try not to worry. He put an arm around around each of us and walked us to the front office. I hardly knew this man, but he had just told me news that would change my life.

We found the car in the parking lot and drove home. We didn't say much. I asked Mom if a tumor was the same as cancer, and she said, "Not always." She asked me how I'd like to go to Hawaii for Christmas. I couldn't believe it. I had been begging to go there for years and suddenly we were going to go. I hoped that I would feel better.

As we walked into the house we found that everything was as usual. The TV was blaring. Dad was making hamburgers for the kids' dinner, and the phone was ringing. But I didn't feel a part of it. Dad asked what the doctor said, and we immediately started crying.

"I have to go to the hospital," I said.

"She has a tumor in her leg," Mom added.

We all had our cry, each for different reasons.

TWO

WHEN I WOKE UP THE NEXT MORNING I WISHED IT were just another day. But it wasn't. I knew I had to go to the hospital for tests. But what type of tests? Would they hurt? Would I have to stay overnight? I'd never been to a hospital even to visit. I thought about the night before. Everyone had acted strangely. Wayne, Annette, and Cheryl didn't fight. I didn't have to do the dishes. And Mom and Dad whispered in their bedroom for a long time. We were even going to Hawaii for Christmas. What was going on?

As much as I wanted to, I couldn't stay in bed forever. Mom was on the phone making baby-sitting arrangements for the kids after school, and Dad had taken the day off from work. We all ate breakfast, got dressed, and left for the thirty-minute ride to the hospital. I made a feeble protest on the way, but my leg hurt too much to put up a very big fight. When we arrived, we went to the Hematology-Oncology Department. We were to ask for Dr. Chard. The hospital was huge, with people milling around everywhere. A nice lady in blue asked if I'd like a wheelchair. I politely said, "No thank you."

"Are you sure? Lots of people here use them," she replied.

Well, I wasn't going to and, besides, I had gotten pretty good at half-limping and half-hopping. Wheelchairs to me were for people who had something really wrong with them and couldn't walk. We wandered through the halls and found the department we were looking for. I saw a lot of small children and their mothers and began to wonder what I was doing at a children's hospital.

Dr. Chard introduced himself and told us Dr. Flashman had been in touch with him and had filled him in on my visit the afternoon before. He wanted me to go to the lab for blood tests, then to X-ray, and return to his office about one o'clock. He was a nice, friendly man—for a doctor. The blood test was awful; I didn't faint, but I came close. I wished I could get over my fear of needles. The X-rays took a long time. The technicians were friendly and helpful. They X-rayed every bone in my body. It didn't hurt but it was exhausting. We returned to the hematology department at 1:00 and I had another examination. I was almost through. All we had to do was wait for the results. I began to relax, and thought, This is almost over and it hasn't been so bad. I was even getting hungry and thought a hamburger would taste awfully good on the way home. There was a football game that night and, although I wouldn't be able to march with the drill team, I thought I'd like to go anyway. Things were looking up.

"Patricia, would you please come into this office?" the doctor asked.

We all sat down, my mom and dad, Dr. Chard, Dr. Flashman (where did he come from?) and myself.

"Patti, it definitely looks like a tumor is causing your pain. We need to find out what kind it is so we can treat it properly. This involves a procedure called a 'biopsy.' Have you ever heard of that?"

"No," I answered.

"It involves a small operation, and you'll have to stay here a few days. We make an incision in your right leg and take a sample of the tumor to examine. We do this with most people who have tumors. It helps us to know what kind of a tumor it is, and then we can determine what types of medicine to give you to treat it."

I knew I didn't have a choice. I could go home and take aspirin and limp for the rest of my life or get this fixed once and for all. What they were saying made sense, but I didn't want to stay.

"I didn't bring a nightgown or a toothbrush, or anything. I can't stay!" I had to put up an argument, no matter how feeble.

"We have all that here for you, and it is important we do this as soon as possible. Come on, I'll have someone show you to your room."

My room was pink, quite cheerful, and I had three roommates around my own age. Janet had been in a car accident, Katie had fallen off a horse and hurt her back, and Louise had been born with a birth defect and was in for one of several operations. They were friendly and not feeling too bad. Our ward was called the "teenage floor." It had a pool table, color TV, stereo, and other things to keep us from getting bored. The younger children were on another ward.

The nurses were all nice. They explained everything that was going to happen the next day. I felt less anxious when Dr. Chard came by my room and answered more questions. He told me that all my X-rays looked good and there was no evidence of a tumor anywhere else in my body. I knew that was good news—but, at the time, I didn't realize how good.

My parents left that evening, reassuring me that they would be back in the morning before surgery. I decided to take a walk up and down the hall. I'd never known anyone sick enough to come to a hospital before. I began to wonder what was wrong with everyone. Suddenly, I felt very glad I just had a growth in my leg. That could be fixed. Some of these people didn't look as if they could be fixed.

THREE

MY HEAD HURT . . . MY BODY ACHED . . . I FELT AS IF I'D
been run over by a car. I was so tired. What were those
things in my arm?

"Patricia, the surgery is over. You're fine. Go back to
sleep," a nurse said.

"I'm so sleepy .. ."

Mom and Dad had come that morning. They were
cheerful and brought flowers and love from my friends.
While I slept, my parents were given the news.

"Mr. and Mrs. Trull. I'm sorry," the doctor told them.
"We got the results from the frozen section of the biopsy
back, and your daughter has a highly malignant tumor
called osteogenic sarcoma. The usual treatment for this
particular disease is to amputate the leg right away in order
to remove the entire bone containing the tumor. It is a very
serious disease, and even with this type of surgery, there's
no guarantee of saving her life. We do know that without
surgery or other treatment, such as radiation or chemotherapy, she probably will not live more than six months. We
have decided to start Patricia on chemotherapy and radiation treatments first to see if she responds. If she does
respond, we will do the amputation in a few months. If she

doesn't then we don't have to put her through a major operation for nothing."

My parents began living a nightmare. My dad recalled his thoughts during this time:

> I was paged to the desk as Dr. Flashman was leaving the hospital. It was pretty obvious from the look on his face that the news was not good. When he broke it to me I think I just kind of went numb and my mind blanked out. I vaguely remember Dr. Flashman being pretty emotionally upset, and he said something like this turned up nearly every year right before Christmas. Your mother came into the lobby about that time, and we had to tell her. Of course, your mother and I were asking about your chances of survival. He could only answer that if you didn't respond to treatments, we might have you for only six months or maybe a year. Dr. Flashman left, and we were in a daze.

The next time I woke up, I felt more human. I had no concept of the time or day, but I knew I had an important question to ask: "Was it a tumor and what kind?"

"Yes," the doctor told me, "it was a tumor, but we won't know what kind for several days. We had to send the tissue samples to another lab to be sure."

The next few days were filled with sleep and pain pills. I went to Physical Therapy to learn how to use crutches. My leg was too sore to put much weight on it. The crutches were to help make walking easier. Friends from school called. They wanted to know what was wrong and when could they come and visit. I told them they could come visit any time and all I knew was I had a tumor in my leg.

I didn't know I had cancer. When my parents found out, they made a decision not to tell me until it was absolutely necessary. If I was going to die in six months, they wanted me to be as happy as I could be during that time. If I was to lose my leg through amputation, they felt they would deal with that when the time came. So I didn't know the tumor was malignant or that the eventual treatment would be amputation. My dad recalled these thoughts:

Your mother and I agreed—one of the few times we have ever so completely agreed on anything—that nothing was to be gained at this point by telling you the truth. Pure and simple, neither of us could go into your room and face you with it. We were completely in shock and had no idea as to the treatments that were to follow or the complexity of the whole situation. I guess we were just hoping it was all a bad dream and that we would wake up with everything being O.K. Maybe the lab people had made a mistake. Hope on top of hope, though I guess inside we knew it was a reality that we had to live with. But, we agreed emphatically to the big lie and proceeded to carry it out. One or both of us should get the Academy Award. Going in to see you that first time was beyond anything words can describe.

I felt better each day and was getting anxious to go home and get ready for Christmas. I became an accomplished crutch walker, and although I didn't like them because they were awkward, crutches were a lot better than a wheelchair. During that week in the hospital, the reality of what was happening began to sink in a little bit each day.

Dr. Chard came by to tell me they were going to start me on chemotherapy drugs.

"What type of drugs?" I asked.

"Two kinds, Patti, alternating each week."

"Each week! How long do I have to take them?"

"We don't know."

"Can I take them by pill?" Please God.

"No, they must be given in your vein."

Oh, shit. "Why?"

"That's the only way these drugs are available and effective."

"Why do I have to take them?"

"To help break up the tumor in your leg. The drugs act to kill the tumor cells."

The next day Dr. Flashman came by to tell me they were going to start me on radiation treatments too.

"What kind of radiation? I learned about that in science, and it can kill you."

"This type of radiation is given in controlled amounts," he said. "It breaks up the tumor and destroys the bad cells."

"Does it hurt?"

"No."

"How long will I have to take these treatments?"

"Three times a week for six weeks to start with, and then we'll see."

The following day the doctors came by to talk about side effects. "What are side effects?" I couldn't stand much more.

"Patti, the chemotherapy treatments may make your hair fall out, you may become nauseated and lose your appetite, your blood counts may drop and you'll have to stay away from people with colds and other viruses. All or none of these things may happen. Each person is an individual and reacts differently. But we have to tell you about the possibilities."

My hair might fall out! Was he joking? Looking at his face, I knew he wasn't. I was only fifteen years old and he was telling me I could go bald in the next few weeks. I cried for the first time since I entered the hospital. I just wanted to go home and forget the whole thing. The doctor told me that he wished there was some other way. When I looked up at him I knew there wasn't. My battle had begun.

FOUR

ONE OF THE HARDEST THINGS FOR ME TO COPE WITH during the next twelve months was that I was *not* in pain. After the biopsy incision healed, my leg felt wonderful. The treatments became worse than the disease. As long as I was hurting it was easier to be cooperative.

After I got my first shot, I was discharged from the hospital and told to return as an outpatient in one week. It was the middle of December and the streets and houses were decorated for the holidays. I didn't feel much in the holiday mood. Mom was four months pregnant and showing. Wayne, Annette, and Cheryl were told the same thing I was about the tumor in my leg: it could be very serious if I didn't take medicines and treatments to break it up and dissolve it, and I would be spending lots of time going to the doctors and they would be with baby-sitters more than usual.

Christmas that year was an unforgettable one. For me it marked a drastic change in my life; I suddenly felt old without wanting to be. For my parents it was unforgettable because they thought it could be my *last* Christmas and our last Christmas as a family. After going to the hospital for my second chemotherapy shot, we left for Hawaii.

The first few weeks of treatments passed. They were not too bad, and I began to enjoy all the attention I was getting from my family and friends. I stayed up to watch the late movies and didn't have to go to school. But once again, reality hit. This was not something temporary; it was going to go on and on and on. Every Monday morning I went to the hospital and had a blood test done and got an injection. I learned not to break into a cold sweat at the sight of a needle but I hated Mondays. To this day, Monday is my least favorite day of the week.

The chemotherapy injections were of two different medicines, alternating weeks. One made my jaws ache like having the mumps. The other made me vomit continuously for twenty-four hours, much like the flu. I called them "jaws week" and "puke week." The medicines' names were vincristine and Cytoxin.

Every other week the doctors would order a chest X-ray. Six months later I found out why they were doing this. The most common place for the type of tumor I had to spread, or "metastasize," was to the lungs. Once this happens, the chance of survival is much less.

I first went to the Swedish Tumor Institute, where I was to receive my radiation treatments, after we returned from Hawaii. I entered a large waiting area that looked a lot like other waiting rooms I'd been in recently and looked around. Many of the people had black lines drawn on different parts of their bodies, lots of them were bald, all of them thin, and I was the only young person in the room. I hated the place immediately. I think it was the baldness that did it to me.

"Patricia Trull," somebody said. "This is Dr. Warner."

"Hi, Patricia. Do you know why you are here?"

"Yes," I said.

"The treatment itself is painless," he explained. "The radiation may cause you to become nauseated, lose your appetite and some weight." (That wouldn't hurt me, I was

24

still ten pounds overweight.) "Your skin will become discolored where the radiation beam will be aimed, and you may lose your hair." Swell. If the chemotherapy didn't do me in the radiation treatments would.

All the doctors and technicians had been briefed that I did not know I had cancer. Lying on the examining table, while they marked my leg with indelible ink, I began to contemplate the whole mess. Was it really possible that three weeks ago I hadn't known a tumor institute or Children's Hospital even existed? They continued to mark the areas they would radiate, telling me I was not to wash the marks off or I would suffer a fate worse than death (no pun intended!). I considered the idea of not taking a bath for six weeks.

The doctors had decided to experiment on me with a technique of radiation that was being used in England with encouraging success. Instead of straight radiation, they would put me into a tube much like the tank they put a diver in when he gets the bends. After I was in the tube, the oxygen level would be increased to four times the amount in the normal atmosphere. This had to be done gradually. It was much like going up in a plane to a cruising altitude of 35,000 feet! The theory behind this method, as I understood it, was the more oxygenated the cells were, the more effective the radiation would be at killing them. It made perfect sense to me, but it ended up being a miserable experience. Every Monday, Wednesday, and Friday I would go to the institute, wait my turn, change into a hospital gown, crawl inside the clear tube, and lie flat on my back, arms at my sides, with only about four inches of space on each side of me and above me. It flashed through my mind that this was like lying in a coffin and once they closed the clear plastic lid there was no way to get out. It gave me a claustrophobic feeling. After the lid was bolted securely over my head, they began increasing the oxygen level, and as the oxygen increased so did my anxiety. My

25

ears would pop and I would swallow madly. I was sure I was going to throw up but knew if I did I would probably drown in my own vomit. It was awful.

There was an intercom system so I could talk to the technician who was increasing the oxygen. Once the correct oxygen level was reached, the tube was wheeled under the large radiation machine. The radiation room was dimly lit. The lethal rays were much stronger than those in a chest X-ray or dental X-rays, so no one was allowed to stay in the room with me while the treatment was given. When the technician had left the room, the steel doors shut and the radiation began. The treatment itself lasted only five minutes, but I had to turn over in the middle of it to radiate the back of my leg which, in the confines of the tube, was a real challenge. After the radiation was finished, the oxygen level was slowly lowered until it was normal. This took about an hour.

I hated going for those treatments and, eventually, the fright was replaced by a strange loneliness. I began to feel like an experiment instead of a person, and as time passed during those six weeks, the treatment became so routine that little was said between myself and the technician. I couldn't tell anyone what it was like; besides, nobody really wanted to know.

Today, this technique is no longer used. It didn't prove to be any more effective than radiation given in the traditional way. But the patient is still alone in the room during the treatment. Closed-circuit television has been installed in many of the treatment rooms so that children can see their parents and the technician while receiving their treatments. They can also talk with them. This seems to help ease many of their fears.

FIVE

IT WAS FEBRUARY, 1968, AND THE SNOW WAS FALLING. I loved winter. The smell of burning wood in a fireplace, and being inside looking out while the rest of the world was freezing. Most of all winter meant skiing. I had never been Winter Olympic material but I sure did like skiing. It was a popular sport in Seattle and ski lessons had been offered through the school district from junior high school on. Most of my friends skied, and we found it a great way to spend a Saturday, even if it did mean getting up at six in the morning. We would party on the bus going up, party on the way home, and spend a good part of the day in the lodge—between lessons—flirting! I did a fine snowplow turn and that was all that counted. But this year was different. I didn't ski and I didn't party—I was just plain sick and continued to take the radiation treatments.

The first series of radiation treatments had ended and a second six-week series, three times a week, had begun. Between the two, I was receiving 8,000 rads of radiation total. This second series was administered without the oxygen.

I was tired of walking on crutches; my armpits were always red and sore and my hands were calloused. I continued to see Dr. Flashman, the orthopedic surgeon.

Each time I saw him I would ask, "When can I get off of these crutches?"

His reply was always the same. "Not for a while."

The bone in my leg had been weakened by the radiation, and without crutches I easily could have broken it. Intellectually I understood the problem; emotionally, I threatened to burn the crutches as firewood if things didn't change soon.

I was still not back at school. Between the X-ray treatments and chemotherapy, I didn't feel well enough long enough to make school worthwhile, so a tutor came twice a week. She was a nice lady and someone to talk to besides my mother. My high school friends stopped calling or coming over as much as they used to. We didn't have a whole lot to talk about, but I always wanted to know what was going on at school, who broke up with whom, and what teacher was being obnoxious. But my world had become doctors, medicine, and more doctors. Theirs was still boys, clothes, and Friday nights. A few close friends stuck by me and would take me to the movies or invite me to parties. It was a good feeling to be included even if I usually felt too crummy to go anywhere.

This was also a difficult time for my parents. They couldn't really talk to anyone about their feelings, except each other. They were afraid if they told any of their friends how sick I really was, it would get back to me through another friend or a friend's children. It probably would have been easier for them if I had known the truth. They could have talked about their fears and uncertainties to friends and talked more openly with doctors. As it was, most of the communication and mail from the hospital was routed through my father's office. They lived those months with the knowledge that amputation might be necessary— and I didn't have a clue.

On a Saturday morning in March, I was lying in bed thinking how glad I was my radiation treatments were almost over, when Dad knocked on my door and asked me how old I was.

"You know how old I am. I'm fifteen. Actually, I'm fifteen and a half."

"Well then, get your clothes on," he yelled through the door, "because we're going to get your driver's permit, and then I'm going to give you your first driving lesson."

That was such a great idea! Driving a car was important to me for a couple of reasons. It was something everyone else was doing, and it also meant freedom. Once I got my license, I could drive myself a lot of places.

I used my right foot for the gas and the left one for the brake because my right leg was too weak to lift up and use for both. We headed out for the back roads for the first of many lessons. Dad got a few gray hairs during my lessons, but driving became something I looked forward to and it helped my morale when I was depressed.

Life was getting better. The radiation treatments were over, and I had decided to go back to school part time. Actually, my mother was sending me back to save her sanity; she also felt I needed to spend more time with my friends. I thought I was going so I could pass tenth grade. My mom and I were close, but it had been a strain being together so much during those four months. It is hard enough for a normal adolescent girl and her mother to get along, but we had the added problems of my moodiness and feeling terrible *plus* her pregnancy. I'd say we did quite well at not killing each other during those months.

Spring arrived and I settled into school. Not going to school on Mondays worked out okay. I went to school full time during "jaws week" and part time during "puke week." After vomiting for several hours, it took a few days to start feeling good again. This system worked well because I knew when I would feel bad and could plan my activities around that. The week I got vincristine ("jaws") I made up for the lost time. One week they mixed up the medicines

29

and I ended up being sick when I wasn't supposed to be. I wondered if they'd done this to see if the vomiting was psychological. It destroyed my plans for the week, but ended up being an honest mistake. After that I made them check the drug carefully before they gave it to me!

My veins had gotten progressively worse and harder to find. Instead of one poke to get the needle in, it would take three or four tries. I was bruised and looked like a junkie. I don't think I ever really got over my fear of those needles—I just got used to them. I would make myself think about something else while I prayed they'd get the needle in soon. At times, it would dislodge after it was in the vein, and we would have to start all over again.

One particular visit was exceptionally trying. Mom and I had spent four hours at the clinic getting X-rays, my chemotherapy shot, more X-rays, and waiting to talk to the doctor. We were both hot and tired when we got home, especially Mom who was now nine months pregnant. I went into the kitchen to get myself a cold Coke but as I was carrying it into the living room I dropped it. Something in me just snapped. I couldn't stand my stupid crutches another minute; they were clumsy and awkward, my armpits were sore, and my hands were calloused. I was tired of everything—crutches, doctors, shots, X-rays, trips to the hospital, and no answers to my questions from anybody. I threw my crutches across the room, lay down on the floor, and started crying and kicking my feet. I was like a two-year-old having a temper tantrum, but I didn't care. I had had it!

My mother very calmly stood by and said, "Go ahead and kick and scream. It's what you need to do."

A few minutes later I got up, hopped across the room to get my crutches, blew my nose, dried my eyes, and turned on the TV. I felt better. My situation hadn't changed, but somehow I felt better.

Six months had passed since my first visit to Dr.

Chard—a long six months. I remember saying to Mom and Dad, "I wish I did have cancer instead of just a tumor so I could die and end this misery. At least cancer has an end; this just goes on!"

I'm sure I hurt them terribly when I talked like this, but Mom just said, "Oh, Patti, don't even say such things." We continued to play the game.

I checked my hair each morning to make sure that it was still there. If I had been able, I would have counted each strand every day. Fortunately, it never did all fall out. Having thick ash-blond hair to start with helped because it made the hair I did lose less obvious. Though it lost its luster and shine, at least I had hair. For weeks I lived in fear it was all going to come out while I was sleeping and I'd wake up bald like all the other kids at the clinic. If it was going to happen, at least I wanted to be awake.

When we were first told that my hair could come out, someone suggested that I buy a wig. I didn't like the idea but then I didn't like the idea of being bald either. So, off we went to buy a wig, "just in case." I had always wanted long hair, so we bought a fall, a hairpiece that attaches to your own hair with a comb. We laughed about it later when we realized that if my hair had fallen out there wouldn't have been anything to attach this $75 hairpiece to!

The Hematology-Oncology Clinic had become a familiar place. I had found out that the words meant "clinic for blood diseases and tumors." Many other patients also came for their treatments on Mondays. I got to know a few of the other teenagers well, along with some of the moms and young kids. A lot of the children had leukemia. Sometimes we would talk and socialize; other times we would just sit and wait for our names to be called. If someone didn't come back to the clinic for a few Mondays in a row, it usually meant they were in the hospital or had died. Nobody asked, but everyone seemed to know. I was struggling with trying to understand why a child should have to die.

SIX

BABY TERESA ARRIVED IN MAY. SHE WAS HEALTHY AND thriving. We now had four girls and one boy at the Trull household. Summer vacation was starting soon and with it the promise of sunshine and swimming. I would be sixteen in three-and-a-half months.

As time passed, there had been no sign of the disease spreading. The doctors became more optimistic and began talking with my parents about amputating my leg. I still didn't know about the cancer or the possibility of more surgery. Maybe I knew at the subconscious level—not by anything anyone said, but by what hadn't been said. Dr. Flashman had become a very dear man to me. On my weekly visits, he was supportive and encouraging. Had I been asked a year before if I thought I could ever like a doctor, the answer would have been an unequivocal *No*. He had broken down the barrier, and I had begun to realize that everyone was trying to help me and not intentionally put me through a lot of pain and agony.

Summertime also meant vacation. I was going to California to visit my best friend, Linda. We had grown up together, until she and her family moved to California three years earlier. We had continued our friendship through letters and phone calls and visited each other every summer. Through the years we'd had some crazy times together, beginning with our first day of kindergarten. We had the same birthday, and when we were six we decided we wanted Santa Claus to make us twins for Christmas. That was not an easy one for poor old Santa!

I was to fly to California for a week's visit, between medicines. Before I left, the doctors wanted a chest X-ray and a body scan. They were holding what was called a "tumor conference," and my case was being presented. This was a conference where doctors from all different specialties (radiology, pathology, surgery, and oncology) got together, discussed a case, and made suggestions and decisions. This way, one doctor didn't have to make a decision regarding a patient's treatment.

Dr. Flashman had asked if I could come to the tumor conference before I left on vacation. He said that they would make a decision on what to do next and whether or not to continue the chemotherapy treatments or change them. I thought this meant there might not be any more medicines! My leg didn't hurt, I felt wonderful, my appetite was good, and my hair was still intact. I was still on crutches but thought I might be able to get rid of them too.

What Dr. Flashman had really meant was that they would decide to 1) continue the drugs or change the drugs, 2) do an amputation, or 3) both, since the disease had not spread. Ignorance was bliss.

Dad drove me to the conference on Tuesday, a beautifully clear and sunny day. I was leaving on Friday for my vacation and was I ready. We waited with the other families whose children were being discussed.

"Patti, would you please come in?"

As I walked into the large room filled with people, I noticed that my X-rays were displayed in the front of the room. I wondered what they saw in them. My train of thought was interrupted by two questions: "May we look at your leg?" and "Does it hurt?" I answered yes to the first question and no to the second.

My knee was in a bent position because I had not been

allowed to put any weight on my leg and the muscles had shortened from disuse. One of the doctors asked, "How long has your knee been like this?"

"About three months, since the radiation was stopped," I replied.

My leg, at this time, was a deep brown from hip to knee. This was the field of radiation, and the skin was discolored. It looked strange next to the normal skin tone on my left leg. The skin also felt hard, not soft like the rest of my leg. They had told me that this would all return to normal in time.

The doctors continued to ask more questions.

"Do you have pain anywhere else?"

"No."

"Have you lost weight over the last few months?"

"No, I've gained."

"Do you use your crutches all the time?"

"Yes."

"Okay, that's all. You can wait outside."

I went out and waited for the results. I wished I had a tape recording of what they were saying in that serious room. Dr. Flashman strolled out a few minutes later and sat down next to me.

"Patricia [he always called me Patricia when it was serious], we've decided that it is time to do some surgery on that leg. The tumor did not dissolve and go away with the treatments we gave you as we had hoped. It has not spread to any other part of your body, however, and that is good."

My mind was stuck on the word "surgery." Oh, shit! All I could think about was my last hospitalization. My father knew the word surgery meant amputation. I thought it meant removing the tumor.

"I'm sorry, Dr. Flashman. I can't have the surgery now. I'm going to California." I felt desperate.

"We can do it after you get back," he said.

I decided to buy a one-way ticket.

Just before I was to leave for California, my leg started to swell. The doctor wanted to see me, but I was leaving and that was final. We compromised by having a phone conversation. I promised to keep my leg elevated as much as possible. The only way to do the things I wanted to do and still have my leg elevated was to use a wheelchair. I agreed to use one.

I wish I could say that I stayed in California and lived happily ever after. Unfortunately, being fifteen and not eighteen had its disadvantages. I was given a round-trip ticket and *told* to use it. Linda made plans to return to Seattle with me because my parents felt she'd be good support for me. They were also going to need a baby-sitter during the weeks I was to be in the hospital. I didn't know how they were preparing themselves during the week I was gone for what was ahead. My dad remembers it like this:

There was no way to prepare for this. We just waited and prayed that it would be okay; and that you would understand and accept our motives for how we handled it so far. I think the fact that no spread of the malignancy had been discovered—at that time—gave us encouragement that you would win the battle. We had been told from the start that even if you lived, there was no way to save your leg. This, I believe, drove me up the wall more than knowing you had a life-threatening disease. I simply could not brace myself for the moment when Dr. Flashman was to tell this to you. God must have had plans for the way part of it was broken to you, in the hospital when things got goofed up. I think it was a bit easier that way. One of the biggest reliefs of my life was when you told your mom and me that you appreciated our not telling you the truth. Many people I know thought we were wrong; and when you said, "Thank you, I appreciate these months of anxiety you have spared me," or something to that effect, I could have cried. It made me feel so happy.

I myself chose to ignore the whole idea of surgery. "Out of sight, out of mind" was my philosophy. I think I hoped they'd change their minds by the time I returned home. Once or twice late at night I'd wonder how they would do the surgery if the tumor was in the bone and why they hadn't done it in the beginning. I remembered asking that question earlier, and the answer had been, "We can't remove the tumor without removing the bone." So how were they going to remove the tumor now?

The whole plan was worked out while I was in California. When I returned, I was to go to Children's Hospital (on Monday, naturally!) for one last chest X-ray. If it was still clear, with no evidence that the tumor had spread, Dr. Flashman was to tell me I had cancer and I needed to have my leg amputated to give me the greatest possible chances of survival.

When Linda and I left for the airport her dad seemed very serious. When he kissed me good-bye he took my hand and said, "Patti, know that whatever happens, we love you and we are praying for you." I had never seen Linda's dad so emotional and I'd known him all my life. What was going on? I thought this was all very strange—I was only going to have a small operation.

Mom picked us up at the airport and announced that it was "girls' day out." She had left the baby and the other kids with my dad, so off we went to the movies, the amusement park, lunch on the waterfront, after Sunday Mass at the downtown cathedral. Halfway through the church service I looked over at my mother. She was crying. I had a funny feeling in the pit of my stomach. Mom didn't cry very often, and I hadn't seen her cry since the day we found out I had a tumor. Why was she crying in the middle of church on Sunday with no reason? I didn't ask; I just began to feel very uneasy.

SEVEN

I WOKE UP WITH A START. FOR A MOMENT, I COULDN'T remember where I was. Then I saw Linda sleeping in the other twin bed and remembered I was home and not in California. Oh, God! Today was Monday . . . the Day. The doctors had promised me I wouldn't have to stay at the hospital; they just wanted to talk to me. I'd heard that before and I didn't believe it now. I wanted to go back to sleep and wake up when it was all over. I didn't know what was wrong but I knew something was not right by the way people were behaving.

After breakfast Mom told Linda where all Teresa's things were. Annette, Cheryl, and Wayne were going to stay with friends for the day. I got dressed and then decided that I wasn't going to go. As long as I didn't go, Dr. Flashman couldn't tell me what they were going to do. I announced to my parents: "I'm not going today. The way I feel right now I may never go see Dr. Flashman again."

"Patti, you have to go."

"No I don't, you can't force me."

"Patti, we don't want to force you, we just want you to get well."

"I am well."

I ran to the bathroom and locked myself in. "I'm not going and that's it," I yelled. "I'd rather stay in here and starve to death than go back to that stupid hospital!"

They left me alone. A bathroom wasn't such a bad place to live. I had water and a toilet . . . What more did I need?

My father was upset—not screaming upset—he just didn't know what to do next or how to get me to the doctor's office. My mom knew me. She had spent so much time with me the past months that she knew I was just blowing off steam and that once I got it out of my system I would go. She was right. Deep down I knew I had to go—I just wanted everyone to know that I hated the idea. I was not a complacent child nor could I easily discuss my feelings about what was happening to me. I communicated best by screaming at whomever happened to be handy. I didn't do this with doctors or friends, only with my family. I knew that whatever I did or said they would still love me, even though I pushed it a few times. Thank God they lived through all the anger and the resentment I had bottled up inside.

By one o'clock that afternoon I was tired of living in the bathroom and had made a deal with my parents. Dad and I would go to the hospital for the X-rays and then come home, pick up Mom, and go to Dr. Flashman's office to talk. I wouldn't have to stay at the hospital . . . just have the X-ray and leave. Dad was smoking one cigarette after another and I was biting my nails.

I went to the X-ray Department. During those past eight months I had gotten to know almost everyone in X-ray. I was feeling less upset now, and we were even laughing about something when a technician interrupted. "Patti, when you are through here they want you to go to the Hematology Department."

I thought, But that wasn't part of the agreement. Then they told me that my dad was waiting for me there, and I also felt better knowing that Hematology was *two* floors away from Admissions.

While my father waited for me, he had asked one of the doctors to give me a mild tranquilizer to calm me down. Dad felt I would come totally unglued when we got to Dr. Flashman's office and got the news.

Instead of giving me a tranquilizer, this doctor called me into his office.

"Who are you?" I asked

"I'm the hematology fellow, Dr. Roberts. I started with the service the first of July. Dr. Chard is on vacation for the month."

Children's was a teaching hospital, and a lot of doctors rotated through there. I had been pretty patient about being seen by so many different doctors through the months but now I was getting tired of it. What does this one want? I thought. Another review of my history? He sat down on one side of the desk and asked me if I'd like to sit down. I didn't really want to but I did. What was I doing in an office instead of an examining room? Where was my dad and who was this doctor?

"Patricia, you know you have cancer," the doctor said.

I looked straight at him and said, "I do not. I have a tumor, but I do *not* have cancer." I was sure he had the wrong chart sitting in front of him.

"Yes, you do, Patti. We didn't tell you earlier because your parents didn't want you to know until it was absolutely necessary. Now, that time has come."

What was he saying? Cancer! I could die from cancer!

"Am I going to die?"

"We don't know what is going to happen, Patti. We do know you can't continue to have that tumor in your leg grow and spread to other parts of your body. You are a very lucky person. Most people with this disease die within six months. For you it has been eight months, and things look very good. The problem with this disease is it can spread, or metastasize, to your lungs. If that happens, your chances of survival are very low."

"What is very low?"

"Less than five percent. Patti, remember you are lucky. Your tumor has not done that. We have every hope that you'll be okay. Patricia, because the tumor is in your upper thigh bone, we need to remove the entire bone. Unfortunately, the only way we can do this is to amputate your leg."

"DO WHAT?" I yelled. I looked down at my legs and could hardly see because of the tears. "How high would you have to amputate?"

"All the way to your hip—we have to make sure we get it all."

Where were Mom and Dad? And Dr. Chard? Did they know this? *Dear God! Please help me!* I got up and left the office. Still crying, I walked down and out the front door of the hospital. My mind couldn't absorb anything I had just heard. I sat on a bench, aware that children were laughing, people were coming and going. But it didn't matter. Nothing mattered. I felt as if the world had stopped and I had gotten off. I saw my father coming toward me.

"What's wrong?" he asked.

I just said, "You know what's wrong."

My father didn't know that I had been told or what had happened. He had been waiting for me to come back from X-ray. He asked me to sit there on the bench—he'd be back in a few minutes. When he came back about five minutes later, all he said was, "Let's go home."

I got into the car and felt like I was going to throw up. I cried and Dad talked. He said that he and my mother loved me very much and if one of them could take my place they would. They were proud of how I had handled the last eight months—they knew it hadn't been easy. He then told me that I didn't have to have the operation if I didn't want to. They would never force me into it. It would have to be my decision. I continued to cry.

"Dad . . . Thanks for not telling me any sooner."

We drove up the driveway and Mom was waiting on the front steps. I think it was the first time in her life she'd ever been on time. She wasn't giving me a chance to get out of the car and go through another scene. When she got into the backseat she asked me why I was crying. My father replied, "She knows."

Mom began to cry and then held on to me. "Patti, when this is all over we are going to Australia." Mom always dealt with stress by escaping.

By the time we reached downtown Seattle, the three of us had pulled our act together. I was ready to talk about what was going on. I had a lot of questions. When Dr. Flashman walked into the examining room I began to cry again. He told me that he was sorry and from that moment on he would always tell me the truth about what was going on with my disease.

He then looked at me and said, "Patti, how long do you think you've known?"

"I honestly had no idea this whole time that I have cancer. I figured there was something seriously wrong, but nobody ever let what it was slip. When I sat in the hematology waiting room and listened to mothers talking about their children having cancer, I'd think how lucky I was that my tumor wasn't malignant. I can't believe that I was so blind! I had no idea until today." I cried some more.

The phone rang, and Dr. Flashman became even more serious. "Patricia. Mr. and Mrs. Trull. I'm afraid that I have some more bad news. That was Children's. The X-ray taken this morning showed a tumor in the lower lobe of Patti's right lung. The radiologist could only see one, but they want her right back this afternoon for more X-rays, called tomograms."

I couldn't believe what I was hearing. Not only did I have cancer and need my leg amputated, now I had a tumor in my lung and my chances of survival just blew out the window. I remembered the saying, "God never gives you more than you can bear." Well, He sure pushed me to the limit that day. I was in shock and felt as if I would never move again. Dr. Flashman talked to my parents, but I don't remember anything he said. I just kept thinking, *What am I going to do? What is going to happen next?* At that point I don't think that I felt anything. I couldn't cry . . . or talk . . . or even think about the future. The whole situation was just too much.

We went back to the hospital for the tomograms and then went home. I was exhausted and just wanted to go to bed. Linda met us at the door with Teresa in her arms.

"Hey, I thought you were going to the hospital for an operation," she said.

"I've been there, Linda. I've got leg cancer, lung cancer, I need my leg amputated, and I'm probably going to die. I'm going to bed."

Sleep had always been a good escape for me. I had never lost a night's sleep from worry—from pain, maybe—but not worry. I woke up long enough for dinner, then went back to bed. Friends had been calling and wanted to know how I was. They thought I was in the hospital. All they were told was that I was home and not in the hospital and would talk to them the next day. I didn't want to talk to anyone; I just wanted to sleep.

Later that night I woke up and again began to wonder what was next. The doctors were having another tumor conference to decide if they should go ahead with surgery, try more chemotherapy, or leave me alone. It all depended on how many lesions were in my lungs.

I got up and played with Teresa for a while. She was two months old and a good distraction for me. I enjoyed feeding and rocking her. Mom came in and told me that the hospital had called earlier. They had decided to give me ten weeks of a new type of chemotherapy drug. I would only have to take it every other week (five doses). I was lucky because the X-ray had shown only one lesion. They wouldn't do any surgery on my leg until they knew if they could control the tumor in my lung.

I was ecstatic! *Time!* I had just bought ten weeks—two-and-a-half months of *time* before they would even consider amputating my leg. For a fifteen-year-old, losing a leg is a very real thing—dying is not. What a deal. A shot only every other week. I hadn't had a shot-free week in ages.

We tried to make the most of those ten weeks. We had a month before school started, so we rented a beach house and packed everyone and everything up for a few weeks' vacation. Linda stayed a while, but then went home after reassuring me everything was going to be just fine. She was mostly trying to reassure herself. The new medicine didn't bother me and I had no side effects. The worst part was just trying to get it into my veins. I didn't tell everyone at school about the possibility of losing my leg, only a few close girl friends. The rest eventually heard it through the grapevine.

I was only seven weeks away from my sixteenth birthday, so I was busy practicing my driving. No matter what, I was going to get my license.

Most of the time during those weeks, I just enjoyed life and tried to forget. I was a great denier, and that was how I coped. I couldn't dwell on the bad things because I knew the problems weren't going to go away. I also knew that thinking about them didn't help me. When something tragic happens or someone dies you feel like everyone should stop and feel your sadness too. But life goes on and you either go with it or you stop living—and I didn't want to stop living.

EIGHT

"HAPPY BIRTHDAY TO YOU . . . HAPPY BIRTHDAY TO YOU
. . . happy birthday, dear Patti . . .!" I was sixteen. Only
four more weeks before the treatments were over and my
time would be up. I got my driver's license, and some of my
friends came over for a birthday dinner. It was a nice party,
but I couldn't help thinking: This is my "sweet sixteen"
birthday and I should be getting kissed by a boyfriend or
having a wild party. I hadn't thought much about boys or
dating this last year. I hadn't really missed it except on
special occasions like this. I wished I could erase the last
year and be a normal, healthy, crazy, pain-in-the-butt,
sixteen-year-old kid.

One of my gifts was a television set, and Wayne and my
sisters had a fit.

"She gets everything; we don't get anything."

"Why are you so nice to Patti and why doesn't she have
to do the dishes?"

The last year was beginning to take its toll on them too.

It was the middle of October and "zero" day had arrived.
My last treatment was over. The tumor in my lung had not
gone away but it hadn't grown or spread either. The

doctors decided to watch it for a couple of weeks—without any chemotherapy—to see if it remained stable. If it did they would do lung surgery and try to remove the tumor. That was fine with me because that meant more *time*.

I saw Dr. Flashman regularly, and he watched my leg closely. The treated area was still hard and my knee was still in a bent position. My foot had begun to tingle and was numb in parts, but there was no pain. I even went to school five hours a day, carrying my books in a backpack because I was on crutches.

We made an appointment with the doctor who would perform the lung surgery. He was a nice man and he was honest with me. He explained what the operation would involve. He also told me that he couldn't give any guarantees. Even with the surgery, the tumor could come back within a month. There was also the possibility that he would find more tumors than the one that showed up on the X-ray. The surgery would have to be my decision. It would not be easy, and I would be in the hospital at least two weeks, and there would be a twelve-inch scar from my side up my back. I told him I'd go home and think about it and call him back.

Meanwhile, something totally unexpected happened. Dr. Flashman died from a freak accident. I just couldn't believe it when I went for my appointment that week and he was dead. His nurse told me he had been at his farm over the weekend and had hit his leg on a tractor, causing a blood clot. The clot traveled up to his lungs, killing him within a few hours. I couldn't help feeling how fragile and temporary life really is. Here I'd been fighting a battle for my life for almost a year and Dr. Flashman's life was wiped out in a weekend.

I felt sorry for his family, but I also felt sorry for *me*. I was angry that he died when I needed him. It had taken months to learn to trust him and believe in him as a doctor, and now he was gone. Who was going to make the decisions about my treatments? Who was I going to yell at when I was tired of walking on crutches? And most important, who was going to do any surgery I might need to make me better?

How many times had Dr. Flashman said, "Patti, you are not in this fight alone. We are in it together and we will get through it together." Now there was no more together. Life was unfair and I didn't understand any of it. I was going to miss him . . . a lot.

I moped around the house for a couple of days thinking about the lung surgery. The subject hadn't been discussed since we left the surgeon's office. My parents had said, "Patti, we would like you to have the surgery, but you are the one who will have to go through it, so the decision is yours." After that they dropped it. I had decided in the surgeon's office to have the surgery but I didn't tell anyone then. I thought I'd exercise some obnoxious adolescent control and just let everyone wonder for a few days. It was one of the few things I felt I had any control over. I knew that not having the surgery would be like quitting and I was never a quitter.

We arranged for the lung surgery to be done in two weeks. In the meantime, my leg was beginning to hurt and was swelling. Since Dr. Flashman's death I had been seeing his partner, Dr. Karges. When he examined my leg he thought there was a possibility the tumor was growing and this was causing the pain and swelling. I didn't get upset at the news because, at that point, it was just one more problem to add to the list. The decision was made to take the time allotted for lung surgery and use it to do a biopsy on my leg instead. They needed to determine whether the tumor was active because there would be no point in going through with the lung surgery if the tumor would continue to seed bad cells. I went home and elevated my leg as directed, and began to think about what was behind me and what was ahead. It was then that I truly began to live one day at a time.

I went into the hospital for the biopsy Monday morning. I wasn't frightened. I was only going to have a biopsy and I had had that done before so I knew what to expect. It was the unknown that bothered me. We waited four days for the results.

"No evidence of active tumor. The X-ray treatment appears to have sterilized the tumor." What I had experienced was a local radiation reaction. *Hooray!* I went home for three weeks before returning for lung surgery.

The biopsy incision had been made on radiated skin on the upper back side of my leg. It didn't seem to be healing the way the last biopsy incision had, and it became painful for me to sit for more than ten minutes at a time. I stopped going to school and began to lose weight rapidly. I had never lost my appetite or any weight during all my treatments, so this was strange. Food sounded good, but I would be full after eating only a few bites. This was very unlike me because, even on my worse days, I could usually manage a hamburger, french fries, and a chocolate shake.

I was readmitted to the hospital for lung surgery three weeks later and twenty pounds lighter. I wasn't happy about being back in the hospital so soon, but I also wanted to get it over with and be home for Christmas. I had been doing my Christmas shopping from a Sears catalog and had strict orders from my brother and sisters: No homemade presents. They were not impressed with all my "recreational therapy" projects.

The night before surgery I talked to a variety of people. The anesthesiologist came by to ask some questions and explain how they would be making me cough and expand my lungs after the surgery, even though I wouldn't want to. It would be painful. The surgeon, whom I hadn't seen since the day in his office weeks earlier, came by. He talked about how I would be in the intensive care unit for several days. Dr. Chard came to say hello. It had gotten to be a bigger ordeal than I had anticipated. That night I dreamed I died.

The operating room was cold, and I was drowsy. There was a needle in my arm, and I was told to count backwards from ten. I knew I would be asleep in seconds and wouldn't remember the time I would lose. I hated the feeling of being out of control. As the anesthetic mask was placed over my face, the ether smelled awful—like nail polish. *Dear God, please let them get all of the tumor out.*

I wasn't sure where I was, but every part of my body hurt. My arms were strapped down, and bottles of intravenous fluid were hanging over me. I could hear the heart monitor going *beep, beep, beep.* Someone put an X-ray plate under me, and it hurt to breathe. *Am I alive or is this hell? I* thought. A nurse gave me a shot and I welcomed the sleep.

The next six days in intensive care were a fog of pain, faces, and more pain. I never realized how much you used your lungs. When I breathed, ate, talked, laughed, or cried, the pain was terrible. Telling jokes was forbidden. I talked and ate very little and would have quit breathing altogether if they had let me. Unfortunately, the therapist came several times a day to make me breathe deeply and cough.

On the positive side, the news was good. They had found only one isolated tumor in my right lung and were able to remove it. The doctors felt confident they had gotten it all. That left me with one question for the surgeon. "Since you have removed the tumor from my lung and found no evidence of the tumor in my leg three weeks ago, do I still have to have an amputation?"

The answer was No! I could have put up with any amount of pain to hear that. I got steadily stronger, breathing became less painful, and I was sent home two days before Christmas. That was the best Christmas present, ever.

48

It was Teresa's first Christmas and a much happier one for all of us than the year before. I spent most of my time lying down. I couldn't use my crutches because they pulled on the stitches under my arm and up my back. Sitting up or being in a wheelchair for a long time was painful. The stitches in my leg had been removed, but the biopsy incision had still not healed. It was draining and sore. My spirits were good, but my body was a wreck. I had stopped losing weight, though, and that was encouraging.

New Year's eve arrived along with ten inches of snow. The new year, 1969, promised to be a much better year. I was anxious to get back to school and see everyone. But as I was recovering from the lung surgery, my leg began to hurt more and more. As the days passed I became extremely uncomfortable, and oral medication didn't control the pain for more than a few hours at a time. I was counting the minutes between pain pills. Sleep became sporadic, and the nights long and lonely.

My mom became my nurse. The open five-inch hole from the incision in my leg had not healed and needed to be cleaned with peroxide daily and packed with gauze. It was a difficult job that required a strong stomach. Mom did this for me so I wouldn't have to be readmitted to the hospital again. It was a gift of love.

The pain kept getting worse. I tried pink pills, red pills, green pills, yellow pills, orange pills, wine, meditation—the effect was short with each. I would have given marijuana a try if I'd known about it. Lying awake nights, I'd wonder how everyone else could sleep while I hurt so badly day after day, night after night. The nights were the worst. I wanted someone to talk to, to play cards with—anything to distract my mind from the pain. The TV went off the air at 1:00 A.M. I would let my mind wander and remember all the fun things I used to do and pretend I was swimming or skiing or at a school dance. That distracted me for short periods of time, but usually I ended up more depressed and

49

full of questions. Why did this have to happen to me? Over and over I would ask myself that question but there was never any answer. I only knew that my family and friends were all walking, active, and feeling good and I was miserable. When would it end?

The doctors suggested my returning to the hospital in the middle of January. I said No. Finally the pain became too much and no distractions helped. On February 2, 1969, one month after the pain had started again, I agreed to go to the hospital. Once again I hated the idea, but the promise of pain control and sleep was stronger than I was. I was tired. Everyone was tired.

NINE

MORPHINE. WHAT A WONDERFUL DRUG. I COULD SLEEP again, the pain was gone and I felt terrific. Even though the morphine could only be administered through an I.V. or shot, I didn't care. It worked. I was in a private room because of the open, draining area on my leg. They didn't want me infecting other patients with staph germs. One South had become a familiar place after three admissions in three months. Feeling comfortable, I thought how nice it was not to be there for surgery but only for relief of pain, and that was definitely being accomplished.

A week passed and the shots of morphine continued. Dr. Thorne, a new doctor, came by to examine me. He was a plastic surgeon, and on Friday he sat down to talk. "Patti, you have a five-inch-long gaping hole in the back of your leg that goes to the bare bone. It is not going to heal by itself and needs to be cleaned out surgically. We hope it will then heal from the inside out. It looks like a large necrotic ulcer and it is what is causing you so much discomfort. Cleaning it out will mean another trip to surgery and another anesthetic because it would be too painful to do while you were awake." It was painful enough when the nurses cleaned and packed the incision once a day, so I gladly agreed to an anesthetic.

51

My family visited me every day. Mom got a sitter for Teresa, and the other kids were in school. She would come in the morning and leave just before school let out so she could be home when they got home. Dad visited evenings after work and had dinner in the hospital cafeteria (a true sacrifice!). Friends came after school at three. They would tell me how terrible the English test had been, who got caught smoking, and the latest love affairs—the important things in life! I was fortunate that we only lived thirty minutes from the hospital. Many of the other patients I had met were from other parts of Washington or from other states, and their visitors came less frequently.

Dr. Thorne did the "surgical debridement," as he called it. I felt fine when I woke up, not groggy or in pain like after the other surgeries. Recreational Therapy was having a Valentine's party. I was still in isolation and couldn't go, so I had my own party while still high on anesthetic. Everyone had to wear gowns and masks to prevent taking staph germs out of the room. It looked more like a Halloween party.

My family had brought me a present, a heart-shaped charm with a mustard seed inside. The inscription read: "If ye have faith as a grain of mustard seed . . . nothing shall be impossible unto you." Matthew 17:20. My faith was still strong, but I had begun to doubt I would ever feel good again.

Days passed and I had not gotten better. Morphine was not the wonder drug it had been during the first week, and I was requiring a shot every three hours. It became difficult to see visitors because I was either asleep or in pain. The days, once again, became oriented to clock watching and pain shots. Doctors came and went, mostly interns and residents, but nobody talked much. I don't know what I really wanted them to say.

"How are you today?"

"Terrible."

"Is the pain any less?"

"Do dogs fly?"

"Are you angry about what has happened to you?"

"I hurt, I just hurt so bad when the shots wear off. What's happening to me, doctor?"

"Excuse me, Patti, I think I hear my page."

The amount of morphine was increased and the shots were only two hours apart. Dr. Thorne came by more regularly to check the wound.

"Patti, I know you are in pain. Part of the reason is because the necrotic ulcer won't heal. The tumor in your leg could be growing. Your leg is still hard and discolored where the radiation was given. When we did the surgical debridement there was very little bleeding. We tested the reflexes and there was little reaction. I want Dr. Burgess to see you later today. He's an orthopedic surgeon."

Something clicked in my head. Dr. Flashman had mentioned that name many months earlier when he had talked about amputation. Dr. Burgess was to have done the operation. *Why was he coming here?* I couldn't yet face the prospect of losing my leg. I was getting closer, but I wasn't quite ready.

"Patti, I'm Doctor Burgess. I just want to look at your leg."

He was a cheerful man and he certainly didn't look like he was going to give me any bad news. I had learned to tell the "bad-news" doctors from the "good-news" doctors. He examined my leg, talked a few minutes, then left the room.

On Saturday morning I was in the middle of a good morphine sleep when I was awakened by four doctors: Dr. Thorne, Dr. Karges, the intern and the resident.

"Patti, we need to talk to you," Dr. Karges said.

Mom was sitting in a chair in the corner. When did she get here?

"Patti, your leg is not getting better; it will never get any better. We need to do the amputation."

"When?" I seemed so calm.

"Dr. Burgess can do it the end of the week."

I looked over at my mom; she was crying. Irene, a favorite nurse, came in and held us both while we had a good cry. Neither of us had any energy left to be strong for the other.

Once I had my cry I was okay. Although I hoped I wouldn't need the amputation, I had begun, months earlier, to prepare myself mentally in case it ever happened. It wasn't something I consciously did. Once the words had been spoken and the decision made, I could deal with it. The waiting during the next five days was hard. I just wanted to get it over with and get on with living. I was tired of hurting, of being in pain, tired of not being a normal sixteen-year-old. The pain in my leg continued to get worse, but they couldn't increase the morphine if they wanted it to be an effective painkiller after surgery. Everyone was beyond worrying about me becoming addicted to the drug, which was happening. I was miserable.

Dr. Burgess came to see me and explained what the surgery would involve. It would be a difficult operation because of the radiated skin. He would perform what was called a "hip disarticulation" in which the entire femur bone, up to the hip socket, is removed. Yes, I could get an artificial leg, but it would be a while. They hoped the skin would heal after surgery, but it might involve skin grafts from my other leg.

"We are all going to do our best for you, Patti."

Once again I needed to focus on something positive and concrete. I wanted to know what an artificial leg looked like. How did you walk with it? Would it look like a real leg? How did the knee bend? The answers I got ranged from, "You can't tell the difference," to "We'll have another patient come in and show you." I thought that was a great idea.

A few days later a girl with a slight limp walked into my room and introduced herself. Her name was Mary, and she had had an amputation a year earlier. Mary had worn long pants, so I couldn't see the "fake" leg; I didn't feel I knew her well enough to ask if she'd take her pants off. It was reassuring, though, to see she had survived the operation. I had 500 questions to ask. I didn't want to overwhelm her but I asked anyway. "How did you tell your friends? How do the boys react? Can you wear any kind of shoes you want? How long did it take you to learn to walk again?" What I really wanted to ask was, "Should I cancel the surgery?" and "Was it worth it?" But I didn't.

The night before surgery I was anxious. The usual parade of doctors came by to prepare me for the next day. I got a sleeping pill and a blood transfusion that night. I didn't want either. I worried about the pain after the operation. I knew that it probably wouldn't be any worse than what I'd experienced during that last month. I kept remembering how rotten I felt after the lung surgery, and that was just a part of a lung. This was a whole leg they were going to cut off. I thought about my sisters and brother and wondered if they'd still love me with one leg. Would I ever get married? Crazy questions. If I died the questions wouldn't matter, but I was planning to live, and I had to figure out how having one leg was going to affect my life. I wanted to talk to someone about my thoughts and fears. Doctors were helpful, but busy and professional. My parents were supportive, but I couldn't really talk to them because we had all gotten into a role of trying to protect one another. It wasn't healthy, but I knew it would devastate them if I started asking questions the night before surgery about what life was going to be like after this operation.

Mom had left a card on my nightstand before going home

and told me to read it when I had a minute alone. I opened
it and read:

Dear Pat,
   There is so much I want to say to comfort you and I
can't seem to find the right moment or the right words.
I want you to know I love you so much and so does your
father, Wayne, Annette, Cheryl, and even little Teresa.
   God will give you the courage and strength to face
this operation and He will help you afterwards to adjust.
After fourteen months on crutches and so much pain I
want you to accept the artificial leg as your way back
to being so active again. Besides, I need you at home
cooking and baby-sitting!
   And I know how you have suffered and, although I appear
not to notice, I am suffering along with you. Our
little flare-ups are good for both of us, and we know
we don't mean what we say in anger.
   After the operation your spirit may want to give
up because it is going to be hard, but I know you have
lots of guts because you have proven it this last year.
Talk to God in your own way and ask for the strength to
face each day and He will give it to you as He has
given it to me.
   I love you more today than I ever have,

                                        Mother

   It would probably make my story more exciting if I said I
stayed awake all night with anxiety, but I didn't. I slept
fine, except for the usual interruptions, and the next morning I was ready to get the show on the road and over with.
The five-day wait had been the torture. I think it was much
harder on my family, friends, and even nurses and doctors
than it was on me that morning. Right before I was put
under the anesthetic one of the doctors asked me what I was

thinking. Groggily, I answered, "I'm thinking about what it's going to be like to wake up and only have one leg—or if I really want to wake up at all."

"Patricia. Patricia. It's over. Go back to sleep."

I couldn't move. Tubes were coming out of everywhere and I was getting another transfusion. I was in intensive care.

"Do you hurt? Are you in pain?"

"No, but why didn't they amputate my leg? I can feel it." My right leg felt like it was up in the air. "Please put my leg down."

"Patti, your leg is gone."

"It is not! I can feel it." I opened my eyes and saw my dad standing beside the bed with tears streaming down his cheeks. "Dad, you tell them. I know it is still there; I can feel it."

I went back to sleep for a while. The next time I woke up I again insisted my leg had not been amputated. My favorite nurses from One South came to see how I was. I could see the clock. It was 6:00 P.M. Where did the whole day go?

"Patti, we are going to show you that your leg is gone."

They gently pulled back the covers. They were right; my leg was gone. Lots of bandages, but no leg. I went back to sleep, too tired to cry or talk.

Later I learned that what I had experienced was called "phantom limb pain." The nerves in my leg had been cut but my brain didn't know it. The sensation was a combination of tingling and pain, feeling very much like my leg was still there. Even today, fourteen years later, I still experience these annoying sensations but have learned to ignore them.

The next few days were a combination of pain and sleep—mostly pain. I was moved back to my own room, and my mom and dad took turns camping out with me, on a cot beside my bed. Every few minutes I would grip the rail of the bed and bite my lips. The pain only lasted a short while, and I imagined that it was much like a labor contraction during childbirth. That continued for four or five days, and I was given morphine shots every two hours. *Dear God, when will the pain end?* I truly thought I'd rather die—I was ready. I was no longer afraid of death and at that point I felt it would have been a welcome relief. The doctors reassured me and insisted the pain would ease. They never checked the bandages but they were sure that I was experiencing "phantom limb pain." I knew that it was *not* phantom pain, it was real pain and I was losing my mind. Finally, a week after surgery, I was taken back to the operating room to have the bandages changed under anesthetic. The doctors wanted to see how everything was healing and if I'd need further reconstructive surgery. What they found was an infected surgical site—the cause of my week-long agony. They cleaned the incision, restitched the wound, and started me on more antibiotics.

TEN

REHABILITATION WAS SLOW, AND MY SITUATION WAS not your typical case. The recovery involved more complications than usual, with a staph infection and slow healing. I made one more trip back to surgery in March with the doctors saying if the skin was not healing, they would begin skin grafts. It *was* healing and I began the road home.

The six weeks beginning in early February went by quickly. At times I felt so miserable I didn't care if I ever went home. But as I began to feel better, it became more difficult to be cooperative and pleasant. I was still in isolation because of the infections and couldn't go out of my room; consequently I had cabin fever. A friend once made an astute observation: "A hospital is a great place to be when you're really sick, but once you feel better, it's the *worst* place." My obnoxious behavior was a good indication I was returning to normal. I asked doctors to leave and come back later if they came during a favorite soap opera. I wrote notes to the dietary department inquiring when they were hiring a new cook. I told the recreational therapist I'd done every craft ever invented, and worse yet, I *hated* crafts! I was really unpleasant to my parents. I thought they spent too much time visiting with other patients when they'd come to see me, so they might as well not have come at all. Emotionally, I was definitely ready to be discharged, but not physically. I was glad, however, to see the hospital chaplain, who had become a regular visitor during those past weeks. He never pushed or prodded or wanted anything. He was just a smiling face who came by to say hello. He wasn't big on selling religion but he always asked if I'd like him to say a prayer. I always said Yes because I was afraid to say No.

I went through some hard and awkward times getting used to the idea of having one leg. My balance was off and I was one-sided when sitting and standing. I would look for two slippers instead of one. I'd sit on the toilet and feel sure I was going to fall in. They were small adjustments, but ones I hadn't planned on.

Dr. Thorne, the plastic surgeon, had taken over most of my care. He had done the reconstructive surgery after Dr. Burgess had completed the amputation. Three small areas around the incision were still not healed. Dr. Thorne checked daily to see how I was and to change the dressing. I never looked when he changed the bandages, and as long as they were on I was okay. A week or so before I was ready to go home he announced, "Patti, we can leave the Ace bandages off, everything is healing well. All you need is a few three-by-four-inch gauze pads over these open areas."

"I don't care; I want the bandages left on."

"Patti, you have to look some time and it's not going to get any easier. Besides, it doesn't look bad."

It wasn't his body he was talking about. He left the bandages off and I screamed and yelled at him. I told him to get out of my room. It was the first time I'd really become hysterical at a doctor. Dr. Thorne always seemed to get the unpleasant jobs and he was not someone I ever looked forward to seeing. He later became a good friend.

I didn't look at the amputation site for several days. When I finally did, I cried and thought how terribly ugly it

60

looked. There was nothing there anymore. I knew it was done and I couldn't change it. I wondered if I'd made the right decision.

A few days later, I remarked to Dr. Thorne. "You know, Dr. Thorne, I don't think I really needed to have this amputation. I wasn't in *that* much pain. If we'd waited a couple more weeks my leg might have healed."

His only remark was, "You know, Patti, the human mind is marvelous the way it can forget pain."

After eight weeks the isolation restriction was lifted and I was free to spread my germs anywhere I wanted. It was great to be able to walk up and down the halls on crutches and to talk with other patients, and go to the poolroom. The first time I was somewhat self-conscious, but glad to be out among the living. My friends had continued to visit regularly but had seen me only in bed or sitting in a wheelchair with a blanket over me. I had some real anxiety about what they would think the first time they saw me without a leg. I knew I had to face it and it would be easier at the hospital than at home. One afternoon some of them came by when I was down in the game room shooting pool with another patient. They told me how good it was to see me up, and that if I was well enough to play pool, I was well enough to be in school! Everything went fine. I realized early on that people took their cue from me. If I was relaxed and not upset about being an amputee they wouldn't be either.

I was driving the doctors and nurses crazy asking when I could go home. They compromised and let me go home for a weekend. I was delighted. Real food, a normal bed, no interruptions in the night, no thermometers—life was getting better. It felt strange wearing "real" clothes. I put on my blue jeans and the right leg just hung there. I looked for two socks and two shoes and then realized I needed only one. It was awful, but at least I was going home. The weekend went well, and it was nice to be with my family for more than just a few hours at a time. I ate all my favorite foods, and neighbors and friends came by. Wayne, Annette, and Cheryl treated me like royalty for exactly three hours. After that, we began arguing about television and I was one of them again. Teresa was almost a year old and starting to walk. A neighbor remarked that Teresa and I could learn to walk together. I knew she wasn't being unkind but I just took it wrong and burst into tears. I was weak and more tired than I thought. By Sunday I was ready to go back to the hospital for a rest.

That following Thursday, I was discharged from the hospital for good. My dad recalls some feelings he expressed in a letter to my aunt and uncle in Australia:

I want to tell you something about young folks. I went through World War II and saw lots of death and misery but I have never been up against something like this that you cannot fight. Patti went through more pain and misery than I would have believed the human body could stand. Yet she came out of it in good shape. God gave her the stamina and courage to fight this thing. She in turn conveyed this courage to Betty and me throughout the whole ordeal, or we would not have survived.

We hope and pray that this is the end of it. Medical science cannot give us any answers. We live day by day . . . Patti, Betty and I never know what the future may turn up. The medical people show no optimism (they do this purposely so you don't get your hopes too high), and we just don't know what the future holds. We are just living day by day and enjoying our time together to the fullest. You don't realize how sweet life is until you get into a position like this.

Everything is easier now than it has been, and we feel we have been very lucky.

At that time nothing was said about checkups or more chemotherapy, and I wasn't going to bring the subject up. I went home to start living a normal life again. If the cancer came back, everyone had done his best—including me. I arranged to see Dr. Thorne once a week for a dressing change where the incision was not totally healed.

The first weeks home were a time of adjustment. I was hesitant about going out in public but that was solved the second evening. I was hungry for Chinese food, and my parents suggested we all go out for dinner and get some. (Take home was more what I had in mind.) I put on a dress since I hadn't figured out what to do with my extra pant leg yet. I walked into the restaurant on crutches and felt that people were staring. I wasn't sure whether they were staring at me or the overwhelming sight of the seven of us. Little Teresa, who was almost a year old, sat in a high chair, beating it to death with a spoon and munching on saltines.

As I ate my dinner I became aware of people whispering, and when one elderly couple got up to leave they came by our table and said, "What a beautiful baby." And then, looking straight at me, they said, "God bless you, dear." It was my first experience of what was to come. Many times while walking down a street on my crutches, people would stop me and say things like, "God bless you," or "Whatever happened to such a beautiful girl like you?" or "Did you lose your leg in an accident, dear?" It made me uncomfortable, but I learned to tell the difference between the genuinely sympathetic people and those who were just plain nosy. Each time I went somewhere it became easier, and within a couple of weeks I looked forward to getting out as often as possible.

It was April and, knowing school would be out in six weeks, I decided to wait until the following September to return. I knew that most of the students in my high school were aware that my leg had been amputated, but I just wasn't ready physically or psychologically to go back. I wanted to wait until September when I would have my artificial leg, having learned to walk with it over the summer—I hoped.

During the summer I saw kids from school at the store, the movies, and the beach. No one ever asked any questions, but for some reason it wasn't uncomfortable.

Mom and I spent eight hours one day shopping for a swimsuit that I both liked and thought looked okay. I had never been two-piece bikini material, but having only one leg made buying a swimsuit even more difficult. Finally, after looking in ten different stores, we decided that I would just sew up the one leg and could then wear shorts or a matching skirt over the bottom half of my suit, taking them off at the beach if I felt like it.

The first time I ventured onto the beach was a rare hot day for Seattle. I really wanted a suntan, so off came the shorts—I just didn't care.

Those summer months were a challenge for all of us. I vacillated between being frustrated, sad, depressed, and angry to happy and thankful for being alive. I spent a lot of time trying to figure out ways to do things I'd done before. I now used my left foot for both the brake and gas when I drove the car. I found that I tired more easily, and it was frustrating to have the mental energy, but not the physical energy to do what I wanted to do. It didn't occur to me that I'd had five operations—two of them major—in the last seven months and *should* be tired. I was going on seventeen and I wanted a job like everyone else. I knew it wasn't the right time and, even if it had been, I couldn't think of anything I could do on crutches. Who was going to hire a one-legged teenager with my medical history when there were at least ten healthy ones trying for the same position. I wondered if I would ever have a job.

There were good times that summer too. I was done with the world of doctors and needles. My body had changed but I was still Patti. My feelings, thoughts, ideas, and dreams were unchanged. I intended to live my life, not just exist or be inhibited by other people. I was only sixteen but in many ways I felt like sixty. I had grown up so fast and made decisions many people *never* have to face. I thought about my friends and their "great worries" about Saturday-night dates and how their hair looked. At times I wished I didn't know about the other side of life but I felt the hard part was behind me and I was ready to go on.

ELEVEN

MY BODY WAS HEALED AND I WAS TO BE FITTED WITH an artificial leg. Dr. Burgess, the surgeon, wanted to see me.

"Patti, you look terrific! I think it's time to get you a limb. A person called a prosthetist will make it for you. Come back and see me when it is finished."

Well, that was what I'd been waiting to hear. It had been almost a full year since the amputation; it had taken that long for the amputation site to heal completely. Unfortunately, I had become so accustomed to using crutches, learning to do everything with them, that using a prosthesis was going to be an adjustment.

After weeks of plaster casts and fittings, my artificial leg was completed. I cried. It didn't look like a real leg. It didn't feel like a real leg. And it wasn't shaped like a real leg. Not knowing what to expect, I guess I expected too much. It was made out of wood and had a knee joint that could bend, so that I wouldn't walk stiff legged and could sit or stand. It wasn't the same color as my real leg and it was hard, not soft. When I put on a pair of pants my real leg would fill the left pant leg out and fit properly but because my fake leg was thinner, the pants just hung loosely on the right side. I hated to wear dresses because even with nylons it was obvious I had an artificial leg. The only way I figured I might be able to look "normal" was to wear a dress and knee-high boots, but that wasn't practical six months out of the year.

I learned that the higher the level of amputation the more difficult it is to use an artificial leg. You don't have the muscles to control it or your own knee to stabilize it. Because my entire leg had been amputated, the prosthesis was secured around my waist with a bucket-belt. It was agony. The physical therapist I saw was kind and supportive. She taught me to do sit-ups and exercises to strengthen my stomach and hip muscles, which are the ones that I used to make the artificial leg move. As my muscle strength improved she began to teach me to walk back and forth supporting myself with two handrails called parallel bars. It took hours of practice learning not only to walk, but to use my muscles to bend the knee, to sit down, and to get up when I fell. I was supposed to increase the amount of time I wore my leg each day. Of course, I didn't wear it to bed at night or when I went swimming, and at this point in therapy, if I had had my way I wouldn't have worn it at all! I hated it.

My body was rubbed raw in places from pressure. I had to take the whole prosthesis off every time I wanted to go to the bathroom. *Whoever invented this bucket-belt device had not thought about the activities of daily living—like peeing.* I couldn't drive with my artificial leg on because it had no feeling when I pressed the gas pedal, yet it was in the way when I tried to use my left foot to press it. At school I was much faster walking on crutches than wearing my leg and using a cane. I would put my leg on before I went to therapy, do the exercises, and practice walking for the therapist. She would tell me how wonderfully I was doing and then ask if I was increasing the amount of wearing time. I answered that I was (even though I wasn't) and then went home and took the leg off, ignoring my family's protests. I realized I was hurting no one but myself, but I just didn't like wearing it. I had learned to do everything without it. The main problem was it slowed me down too much.

Whenever I went to Dr. Burgess's office he would ask in a nice but firm way, "How are you doing?"

"Fine."

"And where is your prosthesis?"

"At home."

"What don't you like about it?"

"Everything."

"You know, it is like skiing. The more you practice the easier it will be for you."

I was seventeen and a half and I didn't care. The more everyone talked about the prosthesis the more I hated it. Finally one day I arrived at a decision. I was tired of feeling guilty about not wearing it; I was tired of wearing it to make other people more comfortable. I decided that when I wore my leg it was going to be for me, not my parents, not the physical therapist, not Dr. Burgess, but *me*! I talked with Dr. Thorne later that week. What he said made sense.

"Patti, the leg is supposed to be an asset for you not a hindrance. It should make things easier for you. If it doesn't, don't worry about it. A time or situation may come when you'll want to use it. You may have a job where you need your arms free, or if you have a child you'll probably find it easier to wear it."

I finally liked this man.

I still had to contend with comments such as, "I have a friend who uses an artificial leg and you can't tell the difference when he walks." Usually it turned out that the friend's amputation was at the ankle. One time a lady in a store walked up and offered me the money to purchase an artificial limb, thinking I couldn't afford it. Unfortunately, by not wearing my prosthesis I caused many people to think I had had a recent accident. They asked me, "What happened?" any time, any place. I was usually polite except on days when five or six people asked me the same question.

Summer was over, and I had been accepted into Central University, a small college two hours from home. I had a physical exam, which was required by the school, and found that I was in good health. My X-ray showed no signs of any recurring tumor.

The university was not large, only about 8,000 students. I was in an all-girls dorm, mostly freshmen like myself. My classes were spread all over the campus, and I found myself doing more walking than I ever had before. I would use my artificial leg off and on depending on where I was going. If it was a class far away, I'd use my crutches. Sometimes I could walk with my artificial leg without using my crutches or a cane, but it took a lot of effort.

A girl in my dorm named Laura became a good friend. She confided to me later that at first she thought I had a twin sister. She would see me with two legs, and at other times with one leg and assumed I had a twin. We still laugh about that. It was Laura who probably had the most influence on my attitude during the first year of college. She convinced me that I had to believe in myself before anyone else would—and I could do anything I wanted to if I wanted to do it badly enough. She was and still is a very special friend.

I began swimming again, now that I didn't have an open wound. It wasn't really any different than before, but it did feel strange to kick with only one leg.

I also enrolled in the Jaycee Ski School for Amputees. I had looked forward to my first class so I could meet some other skiers with the same problem, but I was the *only* student! Skiing was tricky. I used one ski and two outriggers, which are basically crutches with ski tips on each. My instructor was an amputee. I spent most of my time learning to side step the mountain, falling down, and learning to get up again. By the end of the lessons, I was skiing and falling a lot, but skiing! It might have been more work than enjoyment, but it was a challenge and it was something I could do without my crutches or prosthesis. I also loved the snow and the fresh air and the chance to participate in an activity "normal" people did. A child in a chair lift once said to me, "Lady, you sure are lucky to have three skis; it's awful hard with only two!"

I had some good male friends my first year of college but I wasn't dating. I was eighteen and self-conscious around boys. I was fine in group activities, but had a hard time on a one-to-one basis. I knew men at eighteen were really into looks and even though I was pretty, I only had one leg. I was so much older than they were in many ways and found myself attracted to the older students who I hoped could see beyond the way I looked. I learned a lot about myself and other people that year. I also learned it didn't matter how much "courage" people thought you had, or how much they "respected" you. It didn't make Friday nights any less lonely when everyone else had dates. However, I firmly believed that, someday, someone would love me for me. Meanwhile I spent my weekends with the other girls in the dorm who didn't have dates. We went to movies, concerts, plays, and all the rest of the student activities. None of us stayed home and vegetated.

Bike riding was a big activity on campus. People rode bicycles to classes and out on the country roads. Every night after dinner many of the students took a five-mile bike ride around "the loop," an area away from the university out in the country. The evenings stayed light a long time, and it was a perfect way to unwind and get some exercise. The first few weeks of spring I waved good-bye as the others took off riding. I had always liked bicycling but I hadn't tried it since the amputation. One day, I saw a used tandem bicycle for sale and thought: I could ride a bike if someone else was helping me pump. Laura was enthusiastic, so we went and tried the tandem out before I bought it. It worked! For many weeks that spring, I enjoyed bike riding. I had to round up a second person to ride with me, but it usually wasn't too difficult. They all claimed I was sitting in the back enjoying the ride and not pedaling! I didn't use my artificial leg when I rode.

As the spring wore on, I got tired of depending on someone else to ride with me. I wanted to take off and go when I felt like it. Laura and her boyfriend suggested I try her ten-speed. She had toe-clips (racing straps) on the pedals, so my foot could stay on. To start, I needed to hold on to a tree or a person while I put my foot in the toe clip. Then I was off. The first time, I was sure I was going to fall flat on my face. Was my balance really good enough to stay on a bicycle? I felt like a five-year-old whose dad has just taken off the training wheels. But it worked and I could ride a bike by myself. I had to stop by putting on the brakes and slowing down next to a tree or pole. At first, I would borrow Laura's bike and go riding with a group of people, not brave enough to go by myself. I needed to get used to starting, stopping, changing gears, pumping up hills. Finally, after a few weeks I decided to venture out on my own. I told Laura if I wasn't back in one hour to call campus patrol—I was probably stuck somewhere. The first few miles were a breeze. Riding a bike was true freedom— no crutches, no prosthesis, just a bicycle and me. The wind blew through my hair, and the fresh air smelled so good. I was riding along confidently when the pedal fell off and so did I. Right into a ditch and the sewer. I was stunned. It all happened so fast I could only lie there for a minute. I pulled the bicycle off the top of me and hoisted myself out of the ditch. I was wet and covered with cold green slime, but the bike was fine, minus one pedal on the side of the road. I felt like screaming, but, instead of reprimanding myself for giving up tandem biking, I screwed the pedal back on and looked around for the nearest tree to balance against in order to start again. It was a good three miles back to campus.

When I got to the dorm I crept in the back door hoping nobody would see me and I jumped in the shower. When Laura came to my room to ask how the ride went, I said that it was fine—until the pedal fell off. She swore that it had never come off before. I wasn't sure I ever wanted to ride a bike again. I did, however, a few days later and since then I've figured out how to start and stop without holding on to anything. To stop I just apply my hand brakes, then put my foot on the ground and hop off. Starting is more difficult but can be done—I just balance without anything for a second and jump on. Sometimes I tie my crutches on the bike if I'm going somewhere and want to get off and walk around. I tie my foot to the pedal with a scarf or a piece of string if I'm using someone else's bike.

TWELVE

IN MY FIRST YEAR AT CENTRAL I HAD TAKEN MANY OF the basic requirements needed to graduate, but in my second year I was pressed to decide what to major in. It was a strange and difficult situation because all I knew was that I wanted to work with children who had cancer, and their families.

Having gone through the experience myself, I had seen many ways a "support" person could have been helpful. Parents sought each other out in the waiting rooms. When their children were in the hospital they visited each other. They were all giving each other informal support, but I felt that getting them together formally would have helped a lot. They could be told, "It's okay, you're normal if sometimes you wish your child would just get better or die." Brothers and sisters of patients often got left out or not told about how their sister or brother was doing. I wanted to start parent groups and sibling groups. Most of all I knew what it felt like to be a teenager with cancer and to have nobody to talk to who wouldn't change the subject or break into tears. All of us with cancer knew who we were, and we'd talk about it among ourselves. At times we needed someone else to talk with—someone to answer our questions honestly.

I wanted to finish college so I could get a degree to work in a hospital and talk with other kids who had cancer—not to tell them how horrible it was, but to let them know they weren't alone and I understood. Anybody could tell you, "I know how awful it is to get these shots, and puke your guts out," but did they really know? When your hair falls out you don't want somebody telling you it will grow back— you want to *see* somebody whose hair had grown back. I wanted to work with children and their families and *show* them that living really was worth putting up with the pain of chemotherapy, radiation, shots, doctors, and surgery.

I had grand ideas, but I wasn't sure what degree I needed or how to prepare for it. As far as I knew, nobody was addressing the needs of the "dying" child or his family members. I wrote to St. Jude's Hospital in Memphis, a hospital for children with leukemia. I thought they must have someone doing what I wanted to do and could give me some direction. I waited anxiously for a return letter. Finally I heard from a nurse practitioner who suggested I get a degree in occupational therapy.

What was occupational therapy? I found that it was not finding jobs for people, as the name implied. It was a field of medicine that gave you a background to work with either emotionally or physically handicapped people. Academically, you studied everything from psychiatry to general medicine and surgery, to normal and abnormal child development, anatomy, physiology, and neurology so that you would have a diverse background and could work with people who had a variety of problems. I learned I could work within a mental institution, a hospital, or a school setting. I could work with children or adults. Therapy involved using crafts, setting up exercise programs, testing to find out a child's developmental level and skills, and so much more. It was a degree with a lot of possibilities; yet it was an area of medicine not well defined.

After I carefully checked it out, I went to some different

hospitals to observe exactly what occupational therapists did. I didn't see any of them working with cancer patients, but was told that they did. Washington University in St. Louis was a highly recommended school for this field. I knew I would have to transfer at the end of my second year because Central University did not have a program in occupational therapy at all. The degree involved four years of college and six to nine months of internship in a psychiatric setting and a hospital. Then you took an exam and became a registered therapist. It meant a lot of hard work, but I wanted to do it. I wrote to Washington University and asked them for their admission requirements and acceptance deadline for the following fall quarter. I also told them I was an amputee and why I was interested in becoming an O.T.

I received a letter stating the admissions date and how happy they would be for me to apply. They would need some letters of recommendation and my transcripts. Washington was a private university and expensive, but my parents said they would help. I began to get excited at the prospect of going to St. Louis. I would miss my friends at Central and my family, but I knew I would be only a four-hour plane ride away. I had my glowing letters of recommendation sent and met all the course requirements to get into the program. My college grades were all A's and B's, so I was sure they wouldn't be a problem.

Now all I had to do was wait. During my Christmas checkup, Dr. Burgess had told me he had a good friend at Washington University Medical Center who could look out for me, not that he anticipated any problems. My last set of X-rays were all good, and I had become his "miracle girl."

Winter came, and I was skiing again and studying hard. Each day I checked the mailbox for a letter from Washington. I didn't apply anywhere else. It was the only school I wanted to go to. There were O.T. schools on the West Coast in California, and there was one in Tacoma, Washington, the University of Puget Sound, but it was a private school and expensive. If I was going to pay for a private school I wanted to go out of state. Finally, a letter arrived, and I rushed to my room where I could be alone to read it.

Dear Ms. Trull,
    We regret to inform you that we cannot accept you into our Occupational Therapy Program here at Washington University. We feel this way due to your medical problems and the distance from our university to your home. We sincerely wish you well in the future.

                                        Admissions Committee

I couldn't believe it. I hadn't had any medical problems for two years and I wasn't on any medication. Besides, the medical school was right there on campus. I was angry and I was hurt. When would people let me forget what had happened? I was trying to build a normal life and I felt healthy and happy. I just wanted to be treated like everyone else. The thought occurred to me that this was a school of occupational therapy I had applied to. Their goal was to rehabilitate a person to the best of his or her ability and help that person lead a normal life. They surely were not practicing what they preached.

After my anger died down I got depressed. I started to ask myself Why? Why even try? Why did I have to get cancer in the first place? Many times before I had asked myself the question "Why?" but never came up with an answer. I continued to question. I thought, Maybe I should just quit school and live off social security. After a couple of hours of self-pity, I went and talked to Laura. We decided I should write a letter to the school and have Dr. Thorne and Dr. Burgess write letters too, stating that my medical problems were stable. We rounded up a couple of our professors to write more letters of recommendation. I wrote a sincere and honest letter and told the Admissions Committee what I thought. First of all, I wanted to know if there was any other reason for refusing me besides a medical one. Then I went on to say I felt the distance between their university and my home should be my problem and not theirs. It took four hours to fly to St. Louis, and it took four-and-one-half hours to drive to many of the universities in my own state. As to medical problems, I didn't have any, and two doctors would be sending letters. I was totally independent on crutches, had lived away from home for two years, and held responsible jobs. I wanted them to reconsider their refusal. A month later I received a simple one-line letter stating, "We see no reason to reconsider our earlier decision. Good luck in the future."

As always, life continued whether I wanted to be a part of it or not. I had now had my first experience with discrimination. I went ahead and applied to the University of Puget Sound in Tacoma, Washington, for the following winter. It was a good school and only an hour from home. I didn't feel much like being an occupational therapist anymore, but I knew I had to do it if I ever wanted to get to work with the kids at the hospitals.

My good friend Patty and I went to Hawaii during that spring break. Patty and I had known each other ever since we started college and had become best friends. Her sense of humor and positive outlook on life were two of the things I enjoyed most about her, along with her love of peanut-butter sandwiches at 2:00 A.M. after studying half the night. Our hotel in Hawaii was right on the ocean, and the agenda of the day was to lie in the sun, swim, drink Blue Hawaiians and go dancing at night. Dancing was a problem for me because many times Patty and I would go to listen to the music and I'd be sitting down and someone would ask me to dance. I'd politely say, "No thank you," and the guy wouldn't pursue it, thinking I was being a snob and not realizing I had one leg and couldn't dance. At times I was just blunt and told him, "No thanks, I only have one leg and don't dance." Most men couldn't handle this, especially at age nineteen, and would get flustered, apologize, and leave rather than just sit down to enjoy the music and talk. It made me feel badly that I was attractive enough to ask to dance but not to sit with and get to know. Looking back, I realize I probably scared guys to death!

On our flight home, Patty and I planned our next trip. We both had jobs for spring quarter and figured that it might be possible to save enough money for a summer trip to Europe. I had a cousin in Germany and I was sure she would let us make our home base with her.

We worked hard that quarter and saved every penny we could. As soon as school was out we planned to be off, with passports and train passes tucked safely away in our backpacks. We didn't know a lira from a mark, but we were going and that was all that counted.

Three weeks before school was out Patty decided not to go. She hadn't saved enough money for the next year and needed to get a summer job. I was disappointed, but understood. I really didn't spend any time wondering what I was going to do. I knew what I would do—I would go to Europe by myself.

I know my parents had some real anxiety about my tripping off to Europe on crutches. But they never said anything except to have a good time. I was nearly twenty and wanted to see as much of the world as I could. One thing I had learned from going through so much at a young age was to do the things I wanted to do and not put them off. Time was precious.

This frequently caused a dilemma for me. I needed to

plan for the future, yet wanted to do everything immediately. Once in a while I would think about what I would do if the cancer came back. Was I using my time the way I really wanted to? The answer was *yes*!

When I first arrived in Germany I went with my cousin to see a castle in Heidelberg. After hours of exploring, I was tired and sat down on the curb while we waited for our bus. Before long, motorists and pedestrians were tossing coins at me. I couldn't figure out what they were doing. My cousin came running over.

"Patti, stand up. They think you are a beggar!"

Although I had my jeans on and carried a small backpack, I didn't think I looked like a begger. After being in Europe a while longer, though, I learned that many people with physical disabilities were beggers. I was shocked! The thought did cross my mind though that if I ever ran out of money during my trip, all I had to do was sit down.

THIRTEEN

IN THE FALL PATTY AND I TRANSFERRED TO THE UNIversity of Puget Sound where we had both been accepted in the occupational therapy program. Our classes—anatomy, physiology, neurology, and child development—were hard and required a lot of memorization.

I had returned to Seattle to see Dr. Burgess for a chest X-ray. Everything was fine, except the area around the stitches on the amputation site had become sore and started to drain. He gave me some antibiotics and told me to come back if it didn't get better.

It didn't get any better but I ignored it for several weeks. I was too busy with school to drive back and forth to Seattle to see him. I did go to the Student Health Center, and the doctor there prescribed more antibiotics and told me to soak the inflamed area in a hot bath four times a day. It was impossible to go to school and take a bath four times a day. I spent most of my time dressing and undressing.

Finally, I went back to Dr. Burgess. The area was draining more and the pain was making it difficult to sit for long periods of time. It was four years after the amputation surgery. It occurred to me that there might be a recurrent tumor at the amputation site. I'm sure it occurred to everyone else too. Dr. Burgess wanted me to go to the hospital. He felt it probably wasn't a tumor but an infection tract. Either way, antibiotics hadn't worked and he needed to do surgery to find out. I went back to Tacoma to talk to Patty. I was upset, and scared, and I couldn't stand the thought of medicines and shots again. Even just going to the hospital after four years would be a hard thing to do.

To make things worse, a good friend of mine, Lisa, whom I'd met when both of us were patients at the hospital, was dying. She had the same disease and amputation I did. The chemotherapy hadn't worked for her and she was at home with her family. I had gone to visit her several times and the last time I saw her she was using oxygen continuously to help her breathe. Driving home I again asked myself, Why? Only this time, Why was I so lucky as to survive? A week before I was to go into the hospital I received a call and was told Lisa had died.

The surgery went well. I hated taking the time off from school and I hated being back in the hospital. Since I was twenty years old, I was too old for Children's Hospital and had to go to another one. The smell of the anesthetic, the needles, the serious faces, all brought back memories of four years earlier. But this visit was short and sweet. After five days I was discharged and the tests had shown no tumor, just a bad infection. *Hooray!* Patty and I drank champagne in our apartment and toasted LIFE!

Time passed quickly. I couldn't remember ever disliking school and studying—it had become a way of life over the last three years. Soon I had less than one year of school left. It was hard to believe.

Before I could be certified as a registered therapist I needed to do six months of internship or work "in the field." I would begin at the Community Psychiatric Clinic in the day treatment program, for three months during the summer, return to school in the fall, and graduate in December.

I had chosen to spend the other three months of my internship at M. D. Anderson Medical Center in Houston, Texas. It was a hospital specifically for cancer patients, with four or five full-time occupational therapists I could observe and learn under. I was getting anxious to get out of school and get going. I had already been working with patients the last couple of years through school. We were required to take a children's clinic, adult clinic, work in a hospital two hours a week, and write chart notes. I had also done some volunteer work at the Children's Hospital the last few summers and had spent vacations working with children who had all types of problems, not just cancer. Hopefully, all of this was going to be helpful when I really went to work.

That spring I took a class on general medicine and surgery. Doctors lectured on different diseases, their treatments, and the modalities we, as therapists, could use most effectively. One late Wednesday afternoon, Patty and I were sitting in the back of the class feeling bored. We were passing notes figuring out what to have for dinner as we starved to death listening to this doctor talk about birth defects. He caught my attention when he began talking about the effects of radiation and the link to birth defects.

He talked not only about fall-out radiation, but therapeutic radiation used in the treatment of cancer. I wondered why no one had ever mentioned to me the possibility of my having abnormal children? I knew I had received a lot of radiation. Could it affect my kids? Could I even have children? Children were important to me. I couldn't envision a life without them. I grew up with three sisters and a brother; kids were just a part of life. My mind returned to the present and the class was over. I confided to Patty that I wondered how much radiation it took to have an effect on unborn children. I decided to go back to the Swedish Tumor Institute where I'd received my radiation treatments and find out. I called and said I'd been a patient there six years before and wanted to talk to a doctor. The receptionist gave me an appointment for the following week.

I was nervous walking back into that building where I'd spent so much time years before. As I glanced around the waiting room, I noticed nothing had changed. My stomach was doing flip-flops and my mouth was dry. I said a silent prayer of thanks for being alive and "cured." I also asked God to give the people in that room the courage they would need to face the days ahead. I was not and never had been an extremely religious person but I was raised a Catholic and believed in God. I believed that everything happens for a reason, or purpose, and though we don't often understand why, we will someday. Until then, you just have to believe God knows what He's doing.

"Patricia, Dr. Warner will see you now."

I walked down the hall into an examining room. I sat and waited, wondering what this man would say. The doctor entered the room carrying a chart, reading as he talked.

"Patti, this is a surprise seeing you." (I didn't know if he meant a surprise seeing me alive or surprise period.) "What can we do for you?"

I explained my concern regarding the radiation I'd received. I wanted to know how much I'd gotten, were my ovaries protected, and what the chances were of having an abnormal child.

"I don't know if I can answer those questions. Actually, we've never had anyone come back and ask."

I found that hard to believe but it was true. "Well," I said, "hasn't anyone ever had a child after radiation therapy?"

"I'm sure they have; I'm just not aware of it except one. We did have a young woman with Hodgkin's disease get pregnant. The child had multiple birth defects. But the woman later had three normal, healthy children. Let me have a conference with some other doctors and get back to you in a few minutes."

I didn't know how they could decide this in a few minutes but I waited.

My stomach hurt and my head ached. I couldn't believe they'd never been asked these questions before. Maybe I should just be grateful for being alive and not ask for any more? But I *wanted* more, I wanted marriage and children, and a career. I wanted to grow old and celebrate birthdays. Why were the things that seemed so natural so difficult?

"Patti, to begin with we think you're probably sterile." *He's got to be kidding! How could he decide that in five minutes?* "You received 8,000 rads of radiation to your right leg. Some of that would have scattered to your right ovary. It also could have affected your left ovary, although not as much. The eggs in your ovaries are there from birth, not reproduced like sperm in the male. So, whatever eggs were damaged by the radiation are still damaged. It could be only a few or a lot. If an egg damaged by radiation is fertilized, your chances of producing a child with birth defects are great. If it is a normal egg, your baby would probably be normal. One of the difficult things is that every woman, radiated or not, has a certain chance of having an abnormal child. Your chances are just increased. And we would never know if a birth defect was due to the radiation treatments or other causes. We don't know for *sure* that you're sterile, but if you're not, our recommendation would be not to produce any children, since we don't know the consequences. There is research being done in this area, but as of now no one knows the answers."

"Can't you do amniocentesis when I'm four months pregnant to detect any problems? Couldn't my right fallopian tube be tied off so the eggs from that ovary couldn't be fertilized?" I knew that, statistically, there was probably very little, if any, scatter radiation to my left ovary.

"I don't know, Patti. When the time comes, you need to talk to your gynecologist. If you'd like another opinion, I'll give you the name of another doctor at the University of

Washington you can talk with. He is studying the effects of radiation. I wish I could tell you more, that I had answers for you, but the truth is, we just don't know."

I thanked him for his time, he wished me well, and I left.

Outside, the sun was shining and it was late afternoon. Laura had gotten married a few months earlier and had invited me to dinner that night. I didn't feel like talking to anyone—I just wanted to walk. I walked up and down the streets and ended up at the cathedral, where I went inside to sit and think. Some small children were playing on the steps and a mother with a new baby was sitting a few rows in front of me. I felt tears trickle down my face. I loved babies and I couldn't even stand to look at them now knowing I probably would never be a mother. I sat there for a long time and thought a lot about the last six years of my life. I thought about how having cancer had affected my life . . . the pain . . . the amputation . . . the uncertainty . . . the discrimination . . . the questions . . . the damage to my self-image . . . the last trip to the hospital . . . and now the possibility of being sterile. Would it never end? I failed to remember the good things that had also occurred.

I knew I didn't really believe I was sterile but I did believe my chances of having an abnormal child were higher. Would it be selfish to take that chance? Hopefully, I would have a supportive husband and we would cross that bridge when we got to it and make the decision together.

I went home and talked with Patty. She loved children as much as I did. She suggested adoption, but I wasn't sure how I felt about that. I began to realize I was thinking about a lot of things that might never happen. I was concerning myself with the future when I had no idea what the future was going to be. I spent a couple of days trying to figure out where this news fit into my life and came to a conclusion: I would deal with it when the time came. Meanwhile, I would go talk to the man at the University of Washington and see my gynecologist.

That summer I started my internship at the Community Psychiatric Clinic. The job involved working with clients who had chronic emotional problems. Many of them had been in the state hospital and day treatment was a stepping-stone to becoming part of the community again. I did one-to-one counseling, organized activity groups, and ran group therapy sessions with the clients.

One of the groups I helped run was called "social group." It met every Wednesday night and its purpose was to get the clients together to socialize. They had lost many of the simple skills we take for granted, such as the ability to plan a fun activity, make the arrangements, to carry it through, and not become frightened in a large group of people. I liked social group. It was fun and the clients did most of the organizing. I was just around to supervise. I also liked my co-leader, Dick.

I had worked with Dick several Wednesday nights before I realized how attracted I was to him. I admired the way he interacted with the clients and his enjoyment of life and of the work he was doing. I was tired of people who disliked their jobs and were unhappy with their lives, especially when I valued mine so highly. Dick was refreshing and energetic. One Wednesday night after we had taken the clients home in the clinic van he suggested we go have a drink. It sounded like a good idea, and I did want to get to know him better. Our relationship began.

Dick was not your everyday, good-looking "hunk" as we girls called it. I had always been attracted to tall, dark-haired men; Dick was short, blond, blue eyed. But he had a constant zest and enthusiasm for whatever he was doing. I had never known anyone to get so emotional over everything from a football game to a Humphrey Bogart movie.

Interpersonal relationships among the staff were not encouraged, but as the summer went on we grew closer and closer and it became difficult to hide our feelings from the rest of the staff and our clients. After work we would often go out to dinner or a movie, or on those rare long warm summer nights go canoeing on one of Seattle's many lakes. One particular night after a long day of counseling we put on our shorts and took a picnic dinner to the lake. We decided to canoe out to a place called Duck Island, have dinner, and relax. The air was warm but the water was still cold. I began paddling, sitting well balanced—or so I thought—in the front of the canoe. As we paddled, we were laughing about something that had happened earlier that day. We were almost to the island, but I was getting bored so I began taking shallow strokes with my paddle, splashing Dick with the ice-cold water. He yelled and moaned but was a good sport, so I did it again, only this time I lost my balance and flipped myself right out of the canoe, headfirst. It was freezing! As I came to the surface, I heard Dick laughing hysterically. I tried to hoist myself back into the canoe but there was no way to do it without tipping the canoe over, so I had to swim the rest of the way. I was closely followed by a canoe and a man who kept saying, "That's what you get for being smart."

Dick was not only a friend to me but also my first real love. None of the men I had dated before had touched my heart the way Dick did. I often wondered what he saw in me. I knew I was pretty, I knew what I wanted in life and where I was going, and I knew that I had a lot to offer someone both emotionally and intellectually, but I still had a problem knowing he could find all those characteristics in another woman who also had two legs. No matter how many times he told me he loved me, had never known anyone like me, loved my enjoyment of life, I still had a hard time accepting it.

When I had dated other men I often wore my prosthesis because I didn't want them to know I had one leg. I would go through a debate in my mind that if I didn't wear my leg then they would know right away about the "real" me and if I did wear my leg, how would they react when I didn't wear it for swimming, biking, hiking, etc. Dick and I were able to talk about these things, and I soon realized that it didn't matter what I did as long as I was comfortable with myself. It didn't happen overnight, but as time went on I became an advocate of liking yourself for who and what you are.

As we spent more time together, Dick became more involved in my everyday life. He began to learn what it was like to live with one leg. We would often stop at the grocery store on the way home from work; sometimes he pushed the cart, sometimes I did. Inevitably some child would come up and say, "Lady, where is your other leg?" Sometimes I would say it was sick and I left it at the hospital. Other times when I didn't feel like a ten-minute question-and-answer session I would just say I left it at home or an alligator ate it. When I did this, Dick would say, "You shouldn't have told that child that," so I began to tell him that he could explain next time. Within a week he was talking alligators.

Parking spaces for the handicapped were a new thing, and Dick loved them. I hated them! I didn't want to park in one in case someone in a wheelchair or a person new on crutches really needed to use it. Besides, I never thought of myself as handicapped and to park there was admitting it to everyone. Dick thought they were great because you never had to look for a place to park and they were always located close to the store entrance. We had many fights in parking lots, and I always refused to park in the reserved spaces. The one time I gave in was at the Old Seattle world's fair grounds during a Labor Day celebration. There were tons of people and no parking anywhere. Dick suggested we park in the handicapped zone. I said okay, just this once and noticed the sign that said Valid Handicapped Sticker Required—Tow Away Zone. I glanced in the rearview mirror to make sure I still had my sticker and got out of the car. We had a great time riding the carnival rides, eating ·

junk food all day, and listening to a band in the open grassy area. When we dragged our weary bodies back to the car, there was no car. We searched the streets thinking we must have forgotten where we had parked, but still no car. I called the police to find that they had indeed towed my car away. They informed me that my car had no sticker, that I would have to come down to police headquarters, pay a fine, and pick the car up. I laughed to myself and was mad at the same time.

When I told them I was on crutches, they said they would send a police car for me. When the officer arrived he said, "There must be some mistake. They wouldn't have towed your car away, especially if you had a sticker." I said that my sticker was in place and they would see that for themselves. Many apologies and a torn-up ticket later, we headed home. I said, "I am *never* going to park in one of those spots again!" Dick said, "Well, maybe."

Dick and I rarely talked about my cancer. He knew I had had cancer as a teenager and that's how I lost my leg but he didn't know about all the chemotherapy and radiation involved, the side effects, and the possibility of the disease recurring. At least, I didn't think he knew. One day when we were out bike riding and had stopped to take a rest, he said, "Patti, are you ever afraid you might die?" I'm sure my surprise showed but I answered, "Dick, everyone is going to die sometime."

"But for you it's much more real, isn't it."

"Yes, but I don't let myself think about it or I would go crazy. It's just something you learn to live with and, yes, there are moments when it's more real, like when I get a checkup. But usually I just don't think about it."

Dick started then to talk about his feelings for me and how scary it was for him to be totally involved with me because along with that involvement came the fear of losing me. I had thought about those things myself. Was it fair for me to fall in love with someone, and have him love me, only to find that the cancer had come back? Would we be able to make it through together? Would I be abandoned? Would that person be strong and supportive or would he fall apart and wish he had never known me? I always hoped that I would never have to find out the answers to those questions, but now I knew that Dick was thinking about these things too.

As the summer wore on, Dick became more and more important to me. He helped me feel good about my body. I was very awkward at first about my own sexuality, but he helped me to realize that someone could really love me for who I was, and the fact that I had only one leg really didn't matter. I loved being held in his arms and I thrived on the passion we had for each other. My insecurities about my body became less and less and my love for him deeper and deeper.

FOURTEEN

IN THE FALL I MOVED BACK TO MY APARTMENT IN TA-coma but I continued to do volunteer work at the crisis clinic on Monday nights and Dick and I continued to run social group on Wednesday nights at the psychiatric clinic. I also began doing volunteer work with Cancer Lifeline in Seattle, an organization designed to help cancer patients who have questions or are having difficulty coping. Most of the work was done on the telephone by volunteers who had gone through a six-week training session. It operated much like the crisis clinic, and callers included both family members and patients who needed a source of support. With all my volunteer work, school, and seeing Dick, I was moving at a fast pace. I spent a lot of time on the freeway between Seattle and Tacoma, a good forty-five minute drive. The nights I would stay in Seattle, I'd drive back to school in the early morning and stumble into my 8:00 class, where Patty saved me a seat. I soon understood why God gives you so much energy when you're young—you need it!

Graduation was not far away, and for me it was getting harder to think about leaving Dick, but I knew I had to. I wanted to learn all M. D. Anderson had to teach me so I could work with childhood cancer patients. One cold November night Dick and I were sitting in the living room watching the fire and drinking wine.

"Patti, I know you want to work with kids who have cancer, but how do you intend to do it?"

I'd given it a lot of thought. I knew there were a lot of needs, but I didn't know how much had changed in the years since I had been a patient.

"I think I'll talk to Dr. Chard and see what he suggests," I answered.

"Patti, I think you ought to go to Dr. Chard with a plan. You've got to sell him on your idea and the needs you saw."

I'd dreamed of working at Children's Hospital, but I was sure the chances were remote. I didn't have any experience with cancer patients yet, except at Cancer Lifeline.

"Patti, do you believe what you want to do would be truly helpful?"

"Yes!"

"Do you think just anybody could do it? Could a social worker or psychiatrist?"

"Well, I don't think it necessarily has to be someone who has been through it, but it does have to be a person who is comfortable talking about the problems of a chronic illness, about dying, and most important, someone who is not afraid of his or her own mortality."

"Go see Dr. Chard, then, and tell him what you want to do and why. Then do it! Offer to volunteer for a few months if you have to. But you owe it to yourself and to those kids to try."

How I had gone from hating hospitals to wanting to work at one I'd never know. I made an appointment to see Dr. Chard before I left for Houston. I walked down the halls of Children's Hospital looking for the Hematology Department and Dr. Chard's office. Everything had been moved around since I had last been there. I passed the clinic waiting room, and it was filled with children and toys. I felt full of enthusiasm and life and kept remembering Dick's advice.

Dr. Chard sounded surprised to hear from me but was friendly and happy that I had looked him up.

"Patti, it's great to see you! What can I do for you?"

I explained that I was about to finish school and go to M. D. Anderson for three months. I told him I was interested in working with the hematology-oncology patients and the ways I felt an occupational therapist could be helpful. Dr. Chard had been a physical therapist before becoming a doctor, so he understood firsthand the importance of good rehabilitation. I asked about the changes over the last several years in the approach to children with cancer and his department's philosophy.

I found out that kids were usually told their diagnosis right from the beginning and were included in decisions and treatment management. Everything was much more open and honest and there was a lot less anxiety for both the kids and the parents. I threw out my ideas on play therapy with young children, the use of a supportive, nonthreatening person working with the teenagers on a daily basis, my thoughts on parent/sibling/adolescent groups, and the idea of a daily exercise program for the children who were hospitalized.

We talked a while about all the possibilities and agreed I could be helpful to the children and their families, both as a therapist and a person who had gone through the experience of having cancer. The next problem was where to get the money to hire me. Dr. Chard suggested I see Dr. Horning, the director of Rehabilitation Medicine. Since I was an occupational therapist, I would have to be hired under his department.

As I left Dr. Chard's office, he said, "Patti, I hope it works out that you can work with our department. Not everybody can do what you want to do. You are a unique person and could be invaluable to a lot of people. Thanks for coming to see me."

That made me feel great. I would have to find funding, but at least Dr. Chard thought what I wanted to do was beneficial and he supported it—that was half the battle. Many doctors didn't recognize that the psychological impact of an illness was as important as the medical problems. You have to treat the whole person. Dr. Chard and Dr. Hartman, the other director of Hematology-Oncology, had worked in the field of childhood cancer long enough to understand that.

I went to see Dr. Horning in Rehabilitation Medicine. After introducing myself, I told him about my conversation with Dr. Chard. Dr. Horning was also encouraging and enthusiastic, but didn't know how he would get the money to hire an O.T. exclusively for the Hematology-Oncology Department.

I asked if any grants were available or if he would help me write one if we could prove there was a need. We talked more about it and left it that he would see what he could do and that I was to stay in contact with him while I was in Texas. I left Children's that day full of hope that between them, Dr. Horning and Dr. Chard would find a way to hire me.

I left for Houston, on schedule, the day after Christmas. Saying good-bye to Dick was the hardest part. We wouldn't see each other for three months.

My time in Houston was busy between work and exploring the city. I was learning a lot at the hospital and my days were full of working with both adults and children who had cancer. Along with the practical experience, part of each day was spent in the library watching video tapes, reading, and testing my knowledge on the different types of cancer, methods of treatment, and complications. It was a good comprehensive course that would give me some solid background if I got a job at Children's Hospital. I had written to Dr. Horning a couple of times asking if he had any news on funding a position. Nothing yet. My phone bills were high from calling Seattle to talk to Dick and talking to Patty in California.

Finally, it was the end of March and Dick was flying to Houston so he could drive back to Seattle with me. We planned to visit friends in California for a few days on the way home. The day before leaving I got a letter in the mail from Children's. I handed it to Dick to open.

"I can't stand it, you open it. I've finished school and I'm ready to go to work. If they don't find some money soon, I'll have to start applying at other hospitals. Open it. If it's bad news, don't tell me."

He opened the letter and smiled. "You've got the job!"

"I don't—quit kidding me."

"You do!"

"Let me see that letter."

He gave me a big kiss and told me to sit down and he'd read it to me.

Dear Patti,

I wanted to let you know that we do have a position available for you here at Children's Hospital. The Directors of Hematology-Oncology, Dr. Hartman and Dr. Chard, have put you on one of their grants and will be paying your salary. You can start work May 1 at a beginning O.T. salary of $10,700.

Congratulations, and we'll look forward to working with you.

Sincerely,
Dr. Horning

I was ecstatic. I couldn't believe it. I had a job and it was working with the people and at the hospital I wanted. $10,700 seemed like a million dollars—I was going to get paid to do what I had dreamed about doing. That evening I thought about how truly blessed I was. I had good friends, a loving family, Dick was here with me, and I would begin work in four weeks.

FIFTEEN

IT WAS MAY, 1975. I WAS TWENTY-TWO. I'D SPENT THE last month vacationing, visiting friends, looking for an apartment, and going to yard sales to buy furniture. I sat in my new living room thinking how strange it was to be living alone; I was looking forward to the change. Change. Adjustments. Tomorrow would bring a lot of both.

I was going to be working with a whole new group of people with different personalities and I knew my job would be challenging, but depressing at times. Marriage to Dick had crossed my mind, but neither of us was ready for that commitment. We had been dating ever since I got home from Houston and talked about living together, but deep in my heart I just knew something wasn't right. He finally admitted that he had seen someone else while I was gone and, although he loved me, he wasn't ready to commit himself to any permanent relationship. I loved him a lot but knew if either of us had any doubts we shouldn't rush into anything.

I slept restlessly the night before starting my new job and was glad when it was time to get up. It reminded me of the first day of school when I was little, only this wasn't the first day of school. This was the real thing.

I got to work at 8:00 and reported to the Occupational Therapy Department, where I met the other therapists. They were all friendly, showing me where the materials and equipment were kept, where my office was, and where the cafeteria was. I had one big advantage—I knew my way around the hospital. I went to talk with Dr. Horning about how to begin picking up patients. Since Dr. Chard and Dr. Hartman were paying my salary, he suggested I go through them and work mostly with their department, but use Rehabilitation Medicine as the base for my office and supplies. And so I began.

I spent most of those first weeks organizing myself, writing a job description and getting to know my co-workers. I was going to be working closely in a team with a social worker, a nurse, and the hospital chaplain, for the Hematology-Oncology Department. I would go to morning medical rounds with members of the Department to find out which patients were in the hospital, what was wrong with them, who was being admitted and who was being discharged. One day a week we would all meet with a child psychiatrist to discuss problems we were having with children and their families, or problems we were having with ourselves. The longer I worked in the field of cancer the more aware I became that the staff members needed that one hour a week to analyze their own emotional status. Working with children who have cancer is tough stuff. You can't give them a pill and make them better; you can't give them a time frame when it will be over one way or another; you don't have answers for many questions—questions children ask, parents ask, and you ask yourself. Every one of us on that team was a human being and you couldn't be human and not become involved to some degree. For some that involvement was limited, for others it was deep. Seeing a psychiatrist once a week provided an opportunity to alleviate some of the frustrations. Nobody was required to go and it was an informal group.

I soon found that doctors had a difficult time confronting patients when the news was not good—which was too often the case. They found excuses to avoid talking to the kids or their parents, concentrating on test results in a discussion rather than addressing the issue of what those test results meant. Children's was a university-affiliated teaching hospital with lots of young interns and residents rotating through it. They had a particularly difficult time—they had never been faced with having to tell a child he or she could die from a disease. But fortunately, there were many good, caring doctors too, who risked being involved with their patient and would spend hours answering questions, sitting by a patient's bedside offering both medical and emotional support to the child and family. Most physicians could remain objective but there was always a doctor who would become overly involved with a patient. One particular doctor—I called him the "One-Man Band"—was everything to families: physician, minister, funeral director, counselor, and friend. It wasn't always good for the family or the doctor, but I learned to accept that each doctor coped the best he knew how. Some doctors painted an overly optimistic picture to patients to make them feel better, while others were pessimistic so that if they failed to cure the child they felt they had forewarned the family that nothing could be done. I was now seeing things from the other side of the fence.

I spent most of my time with the children. There were usually around ten cancer patients in the hospital at a time, although the number could fluctuate from three to twenty-five at any one time. Nothing was predictable in this field. I think that was one of the reasons I liked it; each day when I went to work I never really knew what to expect. The day could be relatively quiet or it could hold one crisis after another. There was no pattern, no routine—the only thing I could count on, unfortunately, was that there would be patients.

The first few weeks were physically and emotionally exhausting. My body was out of shape and tired quickly from working nine-hour days and walking "miles" through the hospital corridors. I was meeting new families and children every day, and that was emotionally tiring. With the teenagers, I tried to build rapport by getting to know them and letting them know who I was. To the younger children I became known as the "play lady." I'd found playing games and doing arts-and-crafts projects a good way to communicate. Children were much more apt to talk about their fears, questions and feelings while doing a familiar activity than during one of my casual visits.

Therapeutically, I tried to find activities that would make them use their muscles and/or help them vent their frustrations at being hospitalized, like clay projects, wood building, punching bags and ring toss. Candyland and Chutes and Ladders were the all-time favorite games with the five- and six-year-olds, and I never knew it was possible to lose so many times. Puppets were a great tool with children who didn't talk much.

I also gathered equipment from the nurses' station to use for "play and needle" therapy. I would let the children be doctors and I would be the patient. They would pretend to give me shots and take my blood pressure and temperature. They liked being in control and doing to someone else what was being done to them. Typical conversations were:

"Doctor, please don't give me a shot."

"Yes, you have to have it."

"But doctor, I don't want you to put the needle in my arm."

"Hold still, Patti. It's gonna hurt."

"But doctor, I don't feel sick, why do I need this medicine?"

"Just be quiet and hold still. I don't know why you have to have it, but you do, so shut up!"

The role playing told me whether the child understood what was happening to him and why. I would relay this information to a doctor or nurse so that if necessary, he or she could spend more time going over the treatment with the child.

Time was the key. I had the time to do many things that no one else could do. I was not a doctor with procedures, tests, meetings and lectures to attend. I was not a nurse with other patients needing attention. My sole responsibility was these children, and I had the time and flexibility to become a nonthreatening, consistent person in their lives at the hospital. I was on their side and I remained constant. These were advantages and were necessary to make me effective.

Coming home nights exhausted didn't do much for my personal life. Dick was understanding and would suggest a quiet game of backgammon or pool. I'd say I didn't want to play games because I did that for a living. One night I was at his house having dinner. I broke down and cried because a favorite three-year-old had died that afternoon and I had spent most of the day with the family. He gently took me in his arms and said, "Patti, you knew when you took the job kids were going to die."

"I know. But I didn't think they'd *really* die."

As a therapist, my ability to deny things in order to cope was not as strong as it had been as a patient. I still used denial though, in that I never really believed a child was dying. When I worked with a patient I rationalized that the child had a chronic life-threatening illness—he or she might get better forever, temporarily, or never—but right then that child was alive. I don't think I could have done the job I did without a certain amount of denial. However, I didn't "play games" with the kids, and I always answered their questions regarding death honestly and to the best of my ability. But I never took away their hope. Hope was a vital, necessary part of their lives and I never saw anyone die without it. It seemed that they could accept what was happening to them without giving up.

In many ways it was most difficult with the teenagers.

Even though they would be dreadfully sick and medicines failing, they would look at me and say, "I know I'm not doing well, but look at you. You made it and I can too!" I represented hope to both patients and their parents—at times unjustly.

I strongly believed in getting patients out of the hospital as often as possible, even for short periods of time. I was forever paging a doctor to see if I could get a pass for a patient for the afternoon. It wasn't possible with the very sick kids, but usually some of the inpatients were children who were hospitalized for routine chemotherapy, radiation treatments, or adjustments to a prosthesis or wheelchair. With some I was able to go canoeing, visit the zoo, or go for a ride in the hospital van. They got more rehabilitation and exercise paddling a canoe or learning to navigate a wheelchair up and down curbs than in the hospital. It was good for their morale and it gave their parents a break. Once again, I had the time and flexibility to be able to do these things, thanks to understanding directors and hospital administration.

At the hospital you were allowed two weeks' paid vacation a year but couldn't take it until you had worked there at least six months. Exactly two months after starting work I decided I needed a vacation. Six children had died in two weeks, including four teenagers. I went home nights and dreamed of dying children. I knew if I was going to survive in this job I was going to have to change something. I remember holding sobbing mothers in my arms and thinking: *Why, dammit, why? Why do people who want to live so much have to die and the people left behind have to hurt so badly.* I was twenty-two years old and I needed my mother to hold me while I sobbed. I didn't want to know about this part of life, but I was in too deep to want to get out. During those eight weeks I found that what I was doing was important and would have an impact. It didn't matter if I helped make it a little easier for only one person—that one person was important.

I went away for five days and did some serious thinking. I spent the first couple of days trying to forget the children and the hospital. In the next two days I decided to quit and explore other areas of occupational therapy. The last day arrived and I decided I would continue working in Hematology, but I was going to leave my work at the hospital when I left at night. I was going to start doing activities I enjoyed after work instead of coming home and brooding. I knew I had limitations and had to accept that there was only so much I was capable of doing and giving. I was not superhuman, as I wanted to be, and couldn't change the sickness, grief, and sadness, but I could be there when I was needed and try to make it a little easier.

I realized my relationship with Dick was in trouble. I had needed a lot of support those first two months on the job and hadn't been able to, or didn't want to, give a whole lot back in return. The woman he had dated while I was in Houston was rapidly becoming more important in his life than I was. I would wake up in the night alone and wonder what I would do without him and think what a void he would leave if he wasn't part of my life. The more possessive and demanding of his time I got, the more he pulled away from me. He said he loved me but didn't want to spend his life with me. My insecurity manifested itself in crazy thoughts like, You don't want to spend your life with me because I have only one leg. At the time I could only view his pulling away as a personal rejection, but years later we both agree it would never have worked between us. We have remained close friends.

When I returned to work the Monday after my vacation I felt much better about my life and realized it was time to put things into perspective. When working with children who have cancer you tend to think of it as a common illness, like chicken pox or a bad cold, because it's the only thing you see.

A new social worker, Laurie Rudolph, had begun working with our group. She was from Tennessee and a delightful young woman a few years older than I. She had never worked with hematology patients before and didn't know the difference between a red cell, a white cell, or a tumor. She was a talented grant writer and was hired primarily for that skill. She was a good social worker, however, and had lots of experience with people. The families and children loved her enthusiasm and lack of knowledge. If she didn't know what something was, she'd find out. Parents taught her more about cancer than any medical book could have. She became a good friend, and we spent hours together discussing the injustices of life and the ability to find happiness within a life of pain.

Laurie and I became each other's built-in support system. We would laugh when there was nothing to do but cry; we would give each other a morale boost over a piece of pie in the hospital cafeteria at 2:00; we would socialize after work and decide we were masochistic for continuing to work in this field of medicine. It was the camaraderie between friends who understood.

Laurie and I were sitting in the cafeteria one afternoon drinking coffee when she said, "You know, this job evokes weird behavior in people. Last night I went home and all I wanted to do was have Frank make mad, passionate love to me—not even make love, just sex for the sake of sex—and not say anything." Several children had died in the last few days and Laurie had been supporting those parents before, during, and after their child's death. "I just needed to feel alive more than anything!" she said.

SIXTEEN

I CONTINUED WORKING WITH DR. CHARD'S AND DR. Hartman's group for the next two years. I loved my work and got to know almost all the patients. Newly diagnosed children from all over the area were sent to Children's by their home physicians to confirm a diagnosis and begin treatments. I would spend a lot of time with the kids during those first few days, helping them adjust to their disease, the medicines, and the side effects. This involved anything from taking them to a beauty-supply company to buy a wig if they wanted one, to introducing them to another patient with the same disease.

For the children and teenagers who had osteogenic sarcoma and needed an amputation, I would spend many hours answering questions, reassuring them about surgery, and I'd introduce them to the physical therapist who would explain about the artificial limb they would have fitted during surgery.

The treatment for osteogenic sarcoma had changed since I had been a patient. Amputation was now done immediately after the tumor was biopsied and found to be malignant. Chemotherapy drugs were given for at least eighteen months after the amputation and patients were fitted with a temporary artificial leg called a "pylon" while on the operating table and were up in a wheelchair and in physical therapy the day after surgery. They were usually discharged within a week. This approach didn't give them time to be without a leg and become dependent on crutches. With the aid of their crutches they were walking on their temporary artificial leg within a few days, and a permanent leg was made after the amputation site had completely healed. In the meantime they were given a set of exercises to keep their muscles in good shape to help properly control their new prosthesis.

There is no doubt that it was traumatic to learn you had cancer and lose your leg all within a matter of days. This, however, increased the survival rate tremendously. One of the hazards of this approach, however, was that patients were often so absorbed in the fact that they were going to lose their leg and the effect this would have on their life, that it took weeks for them to begin dealing with the fact that they had cancer. I wonder how I would have adjusted if I had had an immediate amputation. It's awfully hard to go from running track to thinking you have a sprained knee to having cancer and having your leg amputated all in a matter of days. New things are being tried all over the country, from bone replacement to using only chemotherapy without any amputation, but the best survival results are still being obtained from immediate amputation followed by eighteen months of chemotherapy.

I tried hard to get patients interested in returning to normal activities as soon as possible, including going back to school. Many times I didn't have to say a lot; just seeing me alive and functioning around the hospital was all most of the patients and their families needed.

One patient, a sixteen-year-old Mexican American named Lester, who found out from his hometown physician that he had osteogenic sarcoma and an amputation was the recommended treatment, came to Children's outpatient clinic to talk to the doctors. Dr. Tom Pendergrass paged me and said he wanted me to talk with Lester. I went to the clinic not knowing what to expect. I walked into a room full of people—eight teenagers and an older man I assumed was Lester's father. Lester had brought his cousins, his friends, and his girl friend with him. He knew he had to make the decision, but he wanted the important people in his life to hear all the facts too.

I introduced myself and his first comment was, "Gee—you're pretty!"

"Thank you," I said. "Just because I have one leg doesn't mean I'm ugly."

It broke the ice and I spent two hours answering at least 600 questions on what it did and didn't mean to have a leg amputated. I gave him my "fight for life" speech and told him that it was worth it. Without the surgery he would probably die within a year—that part had not changed with time. He went home to think about it and decided to go ahead with the surgery.

Lester was a character; he was a teenager you couldn't help but love, as frustrating as he was at times. He protested everything, then went ahead and did it. His surgery went very well.

He began wearing a hat while he still had a head full of hair because he didn't know what he was going to do when it started to fall out. Everyone knew that Lester loved beer even though he was underage. His cousin was getting married one week after Lester's surgery, and Lester said he was "gonna be there." He wasn't going to do a lot of dancing, just drink a lot of beer! And so began the rehabilitation of Lester Recendes.

The first few months, he faithfully arrived for his medicines with a lot of protest and accompanied by his parents. As the year went on, he repeatedly threatened to quit his treatments. On the side I'd say, "Lester, are you serious?" and he'd answer, "No, I just like to shake my mom up!

Besides, Cheryl [his girl friend] won't let me."

He became good friends with many of the nurses and eventually drove himself over from Yakima, two hours away, for his treatments and made it a weekend party. He quit school and took a general education test that allowed him to start college. He got his permanent artificial leg and would periodically drop into Rehabilitation Medicine for us to see him. His gait was terrible when he walked. We had given him some exercises to strengthen the muscles that would help him walk properly, but he didn't care—he hated exercises.

I continued to hassle him to come for more physical therapy, but Lester had a mind of his own. He was a good kid with a great sense of humor and often told me he was going to college to get a degree to do what I did because he couldn't believe anyone would pay me to "shoot the bull!" On his eighteenth birthday we had a party, and he announced that he was now a legal adult and was quitting chemotherapy. He only had six more treatments to go, and we all knew he wouldn't quit. He had too much fun terrorizing us when he came for his medicine. Lester had his bad times—he quit school, ran away for a while, and his girl friend left him temporarily. Most important, though, he continued to live a full and normal life. I saw him recently, three years after his amputation. He proudly walked into the clinic one day and introduced us to his wife, Cheryl, and his new son, little Les. He was off chemotherapy and attending a university. He still walked with a sailor's gait and his hair had grown back curly and he hated it. He was still a rebel and a fighter and was going to live his life to the fullest. He still wants my job.

The teenagers were not the only ones who could handle the truth about their disease. One day I was hurrying down the hall when Kenny, a seven-year-old who had a type of stomach tumor, called to me from his room.

"Hey Patti, come here."

I went in, and he asked what I was doing.

"I'm going to take Marie some paints and paper." I had spent the morning with Kenny making a kite out of straws and tissue paper. We had turned on the fan next to his bed to fly it, and it worked.

"Patti, I just wanted to tell you I might not be seeing you much longer 'cuz the white horse is coming to get me."

Damn!! "The white horse, Kenny. Can I go too?"

"No, Patti, you have to die to go for a ride on the white horse."

"Oh. Are you scared?"

"No. I just wanted to let you know."

"Thanks Kenny." I gave him a hug and told him I'd be back in the morning as usual. When I left his room I thought it odd he chose that time to pull me in out of the hall. I had spent all morning with him and he hadn't said a thing.

I found that children chose their own time, place, and way to tell you what they want you to know. Kenny was not unusually sick from his cancer and just in for routine chemotherapy that required hospitalization. He died three weeks later.

Many times it is as hard on the staff as it is on the patient when things are not going well. One of those times is when the doctors run out of medicines to give a patient. The family and child want to continue to try to control the tumor or leukemia, but there are no more drugs that are effective against that particular type of disease that haven't already been tried. Sometimes the same drug has been given over and over with no improvement in the disease. When this happens, treatment is either stopped or a placebo is given with the parents' consent. The child at that point has usually been through so much, no one, including his family, wants him to suffer anymore. It is a difficult but

109

necessary decision, usually made by the attending doctors. Sometimes there is just nothing more anyone can do. This was the case with a wonderful twelve-year-old boy named Kelly Martin.

Kelly and his twin brother Kerry were the oldest of five children. Kelly had been ill on and off for seven years with lymphoma, a type of cancer of the lymph glands. Much of those seven years he was in remission and felt well. Kelly went to school, he was a Boy Scout, and he was on the swimming team with Kerry.

Whenever Kelly was hospitalized for treatments, his mother, Jan, would room in with him on the pull-out couch. Kelly's father, Bob, kept the house and other four kids running smoothly while Jan and Kelly were away. It was a three-hour drive from their home in Eastern Washington to the hospital, but Bob would often make the trip over with Kelly's brothers and sister on weekends.

In the last year, Kelly had been admitted to the hospital more and more often. His stays were longer, up to two months at a time. The drugs he was receiving to control the lymphoma were no longer effective, and his remissions became shorter and shorter.

In early October he was admitted and put on antibiotics for a bad infection. He was frequently in pain. In spite of this, he continued to want visitors. He liked the recreational therapist to come, and I would visit daily to do exercises, go for a walk, or provide a craft activity.

Halloween arrived, and we bribed dietary for a sharp knife to carve a pumpkin. Kelly was disappointed he wasn't going to get to go trick-or-treating with the other kids at home. I said, "Kelly, you can go trick-or-treating here at the nurses' stations on the different wards."

"Patti, all they give you is sugarless gum and health food, like apples." It hadn't occurred to him that he hadn't eaten anything for days. But, to him, what was Halloween without junk food.

In November, Kelly got progressively weaker. He was in

110

such pain that his mother found it difficult to be around him. For that matter, I did too. One day I walked into his room and he was moaning.

"Kelly, do you feel like doing anything?" I asked him.

"No."

"How about if I read you a book to take your mind off the pain?"

"No."

"Can I just sit here with your mom awhile?"

"Yes."

I sat on the couch not knowing what to do, as he moaned and cried. The pain medication the nurse had given him didn't seem to help. Sometimes when I couldn't help a child all I could do was support the parent. That's what I did that day as I sat with Jan Martin for an hour.

Finally, Kelly said, "Mom, maybe I'd be more comfortable if I moved to the couch."

We would have tried anything. Carefully, we helped him to the couch and laid him down. He began to moan.

"Mom, why does God make little boys hurt so much?"

"I don't know, Kelly."

I looked at Jan—both of us had tears streaming down our faces. I never hurt so badly for another person as I did for her that morning. She was a strong and gutsy lady. I read Kelly a book and he went to sleep. Jan went for a walk. When I saw her later that day I invited her to the mothers' exercise group I had started.

It had begun as a joke. Many of the patients' moms roomed in with their children and complained that all the exercise they got was walking to the cafeteria and back. Their children got more exercise (from me) than they did. So I arranged for them to use the physical-therapy gym, letting them use the exercise bike, wall weights, and floor mats, two evenings a week from 4:30 to 5:30. I also directed some group exercises. This proved a good way to get the mothers together and out of their children's rooms, as well as a way to work out some frustrations.

Naturally, they wanted to know where the music was and why there wasn't any punch to drink. They wanted a high-class health spa. We usually exercised only half the time and talked the other half. It was a fun group of mothers, and you would never have known they had sick kids downstairs, except for the way they half-listened for their names to be paged over the hospital intercom.

We analyzed our fat bodies and swore off hospital food. Sometimes after their kids were all asleep the moms would gather in the ward lounge for a glass of wine and talk. They took turns bringing the wine, and I threatened to cut off their drinks if they didn't "work out" twice a week. Some of those moms were only a few years older than I. How nice it was for me to be able to walk out of that hospital at night. They couldn't leave—their children were fighting a battle that didn't have a lot of winners and they knew it.

Kelly would have good days and bad. He consistently and insistently wanted his daily exercises. It was the bicentennial year, and we were working on a Turkish loom rug of the American flag. I would hand him the yarn and he'd do the Turkish knots. It became important to him to know when I was coming each day so he could plan his naps and pain medicine.

I rarely set a schedule with the patients in case something happened and I couldn't follow through. If a family or child were in a crisis and needed to see me, I didn't like disappointing the child who was waiting for me according to his/her schedule. I found, however, the more out of control and closer to death children got, the more they wanted structure and control. I told Kelly I'd be by each day at 10:00 and 3:00 unless I had an emergency. We made a schedule for him to put on his door with times for his bath, naps, recreational therapy, exercises, bed change, and doctors' visits.

It was mid-November, and he wanted to work on Christmas presents and exercise during the morning session and work on the flag in the afternoon. He was getting more morphine at that point and was feeling extremely good. He was like a miniature drunk and was very funny!

One day we were working on his flag and his mom was getting ready to go have a cup of coffee. She often would leave when I came, as a break for herself and to give Kelly and me time alone. Sometimes children talked much more freely about their concerns and fears about their disease when no parents were around.

Suddenly Kelly said, "Mom, this room is a mess. You have to clean it up. Do you think you're on vacation over here? Do I have to get out of bed and clean it myself?"

Jan and I looked at each other and burst out laughing. Was this the same kid we were crying about a week earlier?

The doctors talked to Jan and Bob, telling them there was nothing more they could do, medically. They wanted to stop the antibiotics even though that meant that Kelly would probably die within forty-eight hours. The Martins agreed, but wanted to bring Kelly's brothers and sister over before the antibiotics were discontinued. They came on a Thursday along with his grandparents. His grandparents were told what was going on and that they would not be allowed in the room if they were going to cry and carry on. His brothers and sister knew he was very sick and might not come home, but not that he wouldn't. Kelly felt great. He was really glad to see everyone. He did, however, send everyone out of the room when I arrived, saying that it was "Patti's time."

I told him we could ignore the schedule that day, but he said, "*No.*"

To go by his room that day, you would have thought they were having a party. I knew his brothers and sister from previous visits and asked them all to come to the activity group I held twice a week. We were doing shrink art. I thought it would give Jan, Bob, Kelly and his grandparents some time alone. I couldn't think about the fact that by this time next week Kelly would be dead. I could only think about all the people who loved him and how alive he was. I knew I was an important person to him and couldn't pull out now, even though at times I couldn't bear knowing he was going to die.

His family left except for his mom and dad. The antibiotics were discontinued on Friday without Kelly's knowledge. He didn't ask why his dad stayed or why I came in to see him that weekend—even though we had a good answer lined up.

Monday morning Kelly Martin was waiting for me as usual at 10:00. We exercised and he told his mom she'd better go to my exercise class that afternoon or she was "gonna get fat."

All that week we worked on the flag and Christmas presents. The flag was almost done, and Thanksgiving was one week away. Late that week a comprehensive-care conference was held with some of the psychiatric interns. They were questioning the appropriateness of this treatment of a "dying child" and who was the crazy therapist who kept making the child do exercises and hook the American flag? I was furious.

"Because a child is 'dying' doesn't mean he stops living. You don't just wake up each morning and wait for it to happen. What Kelly is doing is important to him and gives focus to his days." I wished some of the "experts" would quit reading about appropriate behavior and look at the total person. What was inappropriate for one person or situation was totally appropriate for another.

Kelly lived for eleven days after the antibiotics were stopped. He finished his flag and his Christmas presents. The day before he died was a Saturday, and I came in to spend some time with him while his parents went to lunch. It had taken us two months to get to the point where Kelly could talk about his impending death. He talked about his grandpa and how he wished he could grow up to be like him. He didn't know why some people had to die when they were little. He still didn't know his antibiotics had been stopped, but he knew he was dying. He asked me if his parents knew he wasn't going to live. I told him that they did, and maybe we could all talk about it. He was talking with a morphine drowsiness, but said Yes.

When Jan and Bob returned from lunch, I told them parts of our conversation. Somehow we got started on talking about Kelly when he was younger. Kelly started telling stories about the important events in his life, mostly about his experiences at summer camp. His mom recorded much of the conversation as he relived the highlights of Camp Wonaka. It was an afternoon of love, of sharing an intimate part of the Martins' life, of realizing death was just part of the circle of life.

As I walked past Kelly's empty room Monday morning, there was an ache in my heart—not for his death, but for the joy he had brought into my life the last two months. I was going to miss my 10:00 and 3:00 appointments with a fine twelve-year-old boy.

SEVENTEEN

MY PERSONAL LIFE WAS GOING WELL. I HAD ACHIEVED the ability to be involved with my patients, but go on with my own life as well. It wasn't something that happened overnight; it took a conscious effort. I remember my first Christmas after starting work. I usually loved holidays and being home with my family. That Christmas all I could do was cry. I cried all Christmas day for the families who had recently lost children and were not celebrating together and I cried for the kids I knew wouldn't be with their families the following Christmas. It was crazy, useless and depressing.

My own family thought that I had flipped. My mother kindly suggested that perhaps I'd like to become a travel agent instead of doing hospital work. Each holiday after that became easier, and none were as emotional as that first Christmas. Thank God!

From time to time Laurie and I would go through phases when we were sure that we had cancer. We would be overly tired and know it was leukemia. We went to the lab at least once a month in the beginning for blood tests. Headaches meant a brain tumor, coughing lung cancer. We were each other's best doctor. She was worse than I and if her legs ached at the end of the day she swore she had bone cancer. Luckily we both had the symptoms and knew it was all psychosomatic.

I saw my gynecologist regularly for Pap tests and again discussed the possibility of my sterility. He felt that the radiation had probably not affected me seriously and my chances of having normal children were good. But, like the doctors at the tumor institute, he wasn't able to give me any firm, conclusive answers.

I also saw Dr. Burgess once a year for X-rays and a checkup. It was always a pleasure to see him and catch up on each other's lives. Even after ten years and no signs of recurrent disease, I would still get apprehensive when he did the X-ray, thinking to myself that whatever showed up could change my entire life. The news was always good.

Gradually my need to talk about work lessened. I found it difficult to explain to people what I did for a living anyway, so I usually just said, "I'm an occupational therapist at Children's Hospital." Laurie and I both found that friends really didn't want to hear about our jobs at the hospital. To them it sounded depressing and morbid and the immediate reaction was either to change the subject or make us into saints. Comments such as, "I don't know how you do it" were common. No one ever asked us, "How was work today?" They didn't want to know. It made it lonely at times, but luckily we had each other and the rest of the staff.

What people didn't understand were the positive things these children had to offer and their ability to enjoy and live life in spite of everything. It was something many fifty-year-olds never learned and ten- and fifteen-year-old kids were teaching us.

If anything, my job kept me so aware of how very fragile and tentative human life was that I crammed as much living into my days as possible. I did the children and myself an injustice when I sat around and grieved for them. I took

117

classes at the university, went night skiing in the winter, swam a half mile before work in the mornings, went to parties, and enjoyed bike riding. Nothing very different from the way the rest of the world lived except, I didn't talk about doing things—I did them.

Vacations were important to me. I realized early on that if I was going to "sell" life then I had better believe in it. That was sometimes difficult while working in a world of disease, shots, pain, and dying. I needed time away from my job. I needed to see things, meet people, go places.

Every winter my cousin and her husband invited me for a week of skiing in Colorado. It became a tradition and I looked forward to it.

I will never forget the first trip I made down to Colorado. A few days before I was to leave, my cousin called to arrange a meeting place at the Denver airport. She then casually announced, "Oh, Crazy George is flying out with us too." She went on to tell me that he was a rich bachelor lawyer friend of theirs who loved to ski and she was sure I would like him. As we hung up the phone she said, "And I told him all about you."

The skiing was great that week and "Crazy George" was indeed crazy. He loved to ski—or should I more accurately say, fly—down mountains. What he lacked in form he more than made up for in speed. He was a very outgoing, fun man who lived life to the fullest.

On the third night we were all sitting around the fireplace in our condominium when George announced that he was entering some ski races the next day. We asked him if he had ever raced before, and he replied, "Heck, no! But it looks like fun."

That next morning was clear and sunny. We went with George to the races and cheered him on—to first place! Watching George, I began to realize more than ever that if you never try anything, you never get anything.

As soon as George joined us at the bottom of the

mountain he announced, "Patti, honey, I'm gonna take you to the top. The view is gorgeous and I know you can get down."

I had my doubts—it was a long way up the mountain and an even longer way back down. But after a sandwich and a couple of glasses of wine I felt confident enough to ski down Mt. Everest, so off we went. We took chair lift after chair lift to the top. Our sunny morning weather had left us, and it was cold, snowy, and the view was almost nonexistent. Crazy George patiently instructed me down that mountain, but if I fell 20 times, I fell 200 times! I wanted to kill George for talking me into this.

Four hours after we'd started we spotted the bottom of the mountain. The wine had worn off and so had my enthusiasm for skiing. But I realized that trip down the mountain was the turning point in my skiing career. I knew I would never ski again or else I would go on to great things. I went on.

That following winter my skiing finally clicked. I was handling difficult slopes, moguls, powder snow. My body was tired, sore and black and blue, but I was exhilarated. It had taken years of patience, not only on my part but from all the terrific people like Crazy George who had taken the time to ski with me and encourage me, but at last it felt like skiing again, not work. And at last I could see that it had all been worth it. I felt ready to race Crazy George down the mountain—and *win*.

When I returned home from Colorado I made a decision. I had been working in the field of hematology and serious illness for three years. The work was still challenging and different each day, but I wanted to take a year off to do other things. It was the only job I'd had since graduating from college, and I wanted to travel without a deadline, write a book, sell hamburgers at a fast-food restaurant—do things totally unrelated to my work.

I set my departure date for January, 1979. The hospital

119

had been so understanding about my extended vacations and short leaves-of-absence that I didn't feel I could ask for a year off, so I planned to quit. I didn't say anything to personnel; I just began saving my money. I plunged headlong into that year knowing it would probably be my last working with the terrific kids, their families, and my co-workers whom I'd grown to love and respect.

EIGHTEEN

IT WAS A TYPICAL FRIDAY MORNING, MID-FEBRUARY, 1978, and raining. It was gray outside, and I thought, What a wonderful day it would be to stay in bed all day and read. My head hurt from staying out late the night before. At twenty-five, I wasn't as young as I used to be!

It had been a long week with lots of new patient admissions. Laurie, our social worker, was on vacation so I was picking up the loose ends with families who needed housing or food money while their child was hospitalized for treatments.

Many people didn't realize the expense of having a child with a life-threatening disease. Insurance companies covered most of the medical expenses, but it was the everyday expenses that most family budgets were not prepared to handle. The expense of transportation back and forth to the hospital, renting a motel room or, for a long-term patient's family, renting a house while still paying off a house mortgage in their hometown. Eating in the hospital cafeteria got expensive as did long-distance phone calls to home. Many times when a child was hospitalized for more than a few days at a time, families found themselves running two households. Frequently there was no paycheck coming in because both parents wanted to spend time with their ill child.

It was these expenses that Laurie or I would try to help out with. There were many times that a silent prayer was answered by the American Cancer Society or Leukemia Society, when they were able to supply emergency funds for these families.

The small children were not aware of the expenses incurred by their families but it often weighed heavily on the minds of the teenagers. They would question whether it was worth spending so much money on them when there was a chance that the treatments might fail. To the parents it never mattered. They would sell their homes, car, and all their possessions if there was a chance their child might get well.

After morning rounds I headed for the room of one of our newly diagnosed leukemia patients. Ten-year-old Todd's parents were understandably upset with the news and were worried how he was going to handle it. I spent some time with the family reassuring them that we would all be around to help them through the next few weeks and that the prognosis in childhood leukemia was better than it had ever been. Todd would be able to return to school, participate in his normal activities, and lead a good, productive life, once he was in remission.

Todd was concerned about losing his hair. I approached the subject of getting a wig and he was enthusiastic. A few weeks later we went to the beauty-supply company to purchase one as close to his own hair color and style as possible. Before we went, he decided to shave off his remaining hair since it was falling out in clumps and made his head itch excessively. He compared it to going to a barber who leaves the hair on your face and neck—only it was ten times worse.

We found him a thick, curly wig that looked almost

identical to his own hair, and he was delighted. While he was walking around the store waiting for his mom, a woman remarked, "Young man, you have the most beautiful hair."

He politely said, "Thank you" and chuckled to himself. As he saw the woman going to purchase a bottle of shampoo, he casually walked up to her and said, "Excuse me lady, but I wouldn't buy that shampoo if I were you. Look what it did to me!" With that, he pulled off his wig and showed his bald head. The poor woman nearly had a heart attack.

Todd continued to deal with his lack of hair with a sense of humor. His mother told me that later on that night they ordered some pizza. The delivery man brought the pizza to the door and stated it would be $5.65. Todd promptly removed his wig, where he had put the money, and the delivery man was so shook up he dropped the pizza!

Every child was different and coped with stress in various ways. Todd's sense of humor made things easier for him and his family. Amazingly, most of the patients really didn't mind being bald once they got over the initial shock. Many of them didn't like wearing wigs because they were hot and felt unnatural. Others kept them on twenty-four hours a day. The girls would sometimes wear a scarf and the boys a cap, but often this was done to make other people feel more comfortable.

It was a painful experience for all when a little girl was mistaken for a little boy. One mother solved this by taping a pink ribbon in her daughter's hair. Another got T-shirts printed up that read, "I am a girl!"

Children could be unwittingly cruel to one another. It only took one on the school playground, teasing a child with no hair or a wig, to send him or her home in tears. We tried to prepare the kids to handle some of these situations but usually they managed just fine on their own.

———————

It was late one afternoon, and I had two more children to see on Three South before I went home. One was Aaron, the Candyland champ. He was a bright, outgoing four-and-a-half-year-old who'd had leukemia since he was two. His mother explained to me that Aaron had never known any other way of life and thought all kids went to hospitals to get shots, bone-marrow aspirations and transfusions. He was a delightful little boy who knew every nurse by name, could dial recreational therapy on the telephone, and wouldn't let the doctors out of the room until they promised to return after rounds for a game of Candyland. I dropped by his room and found him sleeping with a Snoopy dog tucked tightly next to him. "Happy Days" was playing on the unwatched television, and the buzzer for the nurse dangled within arm's reach over the rails of the bed. I noticed Aaron's I.V. was not in his hand or arm as usual, but in his foot, the chemotherapy medicine dripping slowly into the vein. I thought about how that would cramp Aaron's style. He was used to getting up, wandering around, playing with other children, and socializing at the nurses' station. I made a mental note to ask Dr. Wilson why they put the I.V. in his foot, but already knew the probable answer. Aaron's veins had gotten more difficult to get an I.V. needle into, and the last time it had taken five pokes in each arm. Not wanting to wake him, I decided to go see Kathy in the room next door.

Kathy was a beautiful, petite, four-year-old ballet dancer with Wilms's tumor, a tumor of the kidney. She loved to have books read to her and knew the exact day and time the library cart came to Three South. I was working with her on an exercise program and encouraging her to take walks a few times a day. Her right kidney had been removed and she hadn't been anxious to get up out of bed and start walking since the surgery. She preferred going for a ride in the wheelchair. We made a compromise: if she would walk with me a certain distance I would give her a ride back to her room in the chair.

Kathy was cooperative; not everyone was like her. Some of the children felt as long as they were in the hospital, why should they have to get up out of bed, get dressed or have the hospital school teacher visit them each day. At times no amount of reasoning had any impact. I have been yelled at, screamed at, and told to get out; I've witnessed hysterics, been almost bitten, and been completely ignored. Exercise time seemed to draw a lot of these responses. Most of the children were cooperative and knew what I was doing was going to help them in the long run. Some of them even looked forward to exercises. It gave them a feeling of, "Hey, I am going to get better and I am going to go home." But for others it was just a chore and a time to demonstrate their anger—usually directing it at me. I learned early on not to take their abuse personally. I've had mothers catch me outside their children's rooms after therapy and say, "He doesn't really mean what he's saying. Please come back again tomorrow."

I always did, but admittedly at times I spent a full morning gearing myself up to enter a hostile child's room, knowing I was going to be screamed and kicked at. I believed in trying different approaches with the kids, including behavior modification, making contracts with them, giving them some control, such as choosing the time I came, and using a reward system ("If we exercise for fifteen minutes I'll also stay another fifteen minutes and play a game with you."). When nothing else worked I didn't hesitate to take the approach, "It's your life and you can lie in that bed forever; your muscles can get weak. Each day you'll feel weaker and dizzier when you try to stand. But it is your life and I can't make you do something you refuse to do. So here is my office number."

I would continue to go by each day to say hi and to tell them to call me when they were ready. It was an "out-on-a-limb" approach, but often enough it worked. Usually these patients had been in the hospital for weeks or months and were sick of everything and everybody—exercising control over *something* was important to them. I found that as they improved medically, so did their attitudes.

It was important to remind myself that each individual coped and handled stress in different ways. When I examined a child's behavior, I usually found that he or she *was* dealing with the illness, just in his or her own way. It was important to look at a child's past coping behavior, before becoming ill. We found that it usually didn't change. If a person had always dealt with problems by keeping them inside, most likely that person was not going to start talking to every doctor, social worker, and nurse who walked into the room.

There are different types of leukemia, some easier to treat than others. Kurt was diagnosed as having one of the most difficult to treat, and the prognosis was poor.

The first time I went to the teenage floor, One South, to meet Kurt, I found a very quiet, introverted young Jewish man. As I grew to know him I recognized that it was difficult for him to talk about his feelings. He was painfully shy. He always welcomed visitors, but being in a hospital and having to communicate with so many people was a new experience for him. He was overwhelmed by all of us—but very polite. His family was supportive and stayed at a motel close to the hospital since they lived about three hours away. Kurt and his family tried hard to grasp what his diagnosis meant, and hoped upon hope that he would achieve a remission.

Kurt was scientifically oriented and took an active interest in his blood-test results and lab tests. I visited Kurt daily and tried to answer any questions he had. I made arrangements for another teenager with leukemia who was doing well to meet him. I also offered him an exercise program to keep his muscles strong while in the hospital and found him eager to participate. He needed something concrete to focus on that would help him help himself because, with his disease, all he could do was wait to see what happened.

Much to everyone's delight Kurt's cancer did go into remission. He returned home where life became more normal. His straight hair grew back curly and he gained weight. He went back to school full time, and as his mother so aptly put it, "It was hard to believe there was anything really wrong with him."

I continued to see Kurt in the clinic when he would come for checkups or therapy. He became progressively more verbal and relaxed.

One year later Kurt had a relapse. Signs of his disease returned, and so began the struggle of more hospitalization, medicines, and transfusions to try for another remission. This was successfully achieved two days before Christmas. Sitting in the cafeteria, his mom said, "Kurt, did you ever think we'd do it?"

He replied, "I never doubted it."

Three weeks later that remission ended, and once again one drug after another was tried. Kurt lived in a state of semiremission for many months. The leukemia cells never totally disappeared but were not numerous enough to destroy all his good blood cells. He watched his blood counts go up and down like a stockbroker watches the exchange. During some of that time he felt well and attended school. Other times he was miserable. One of the drugs he received gave him mouth ulcers, and he could not swallow, talk, or eat without excruciating pain. A friend of his made a pointer board for him with the letters of the alphabet so that he could communicate. The more out of control Kurt's disease became, the more anxious he became. He needed concrete data to concentrate on.

One day he had the doctor draw up a chart of all the drugs known that had any possible effect on cancer. On the other side of the chart he listed all the drugs he had taken. Few remained. We were talking one day, and he said, "You

127

know, Patti, at times I wish I was a Buddhist."

I asked why, and he said, "Because they have such a strong belief in reincarnation. I wouldn't be so afraid to die if I knew what was coming after."

On Kurt's seventeenth birthday, we had a party in his hospital room. He was not doing well, and I couldn't help wondering what Kurt was thinking. Later that weekend he called each member of his family into his room, one at a time. He wanted to tell them what he felt was important in life and what wasn't. This was the same child who two years before could not communicate with his family at all.

He talked a long time with his dad, telling him he worked too hard and needed to spend more time with the family. He also told him that he needed to communicate and let people know what he was thinking and feeling. With his mom, he talked about dying and told her he didn't want her sitting around being sad after he was gone but wanted her to go to parties, like before he was sick, and be happy.

"I don't want you to sit around, turn gray and fat and stay home!"

He talked with his brother about how he should try to get along with their parents. He told Joe, who was eighteen, he no longer felt close like they were as kids and wanted to work on becoming closer to him. Maria, his only and younger sister, he told the important things to know as she grew up. His message was clear to all. Live your life, love one another, and communicate that love.

When I returned to work the next day he shared with me his visits with his family. He looked at me and said with a twinkle in his eye, "Next I'm gonna start working on getting them to touch one another!"

Weeks passed, and Kurt's leukemia remained the same—in limbo. One drug was holding his blood count in a semiremission, but no one knew for how long. Kurt knew his time was short, and it was like waiting for a time bomb to go off. No one knew how, when, or why. He spent as much time at home as possible, but when in the hospital, he would confide to me, "I don't want to die. How can someone who wants to live so much die? I have so many things left I want to do and I want to do something important. I don't want to die and not have done anything significant."

I tried to tell him what he had done for his family and for me was important and significant. Kurt truly lived until the day he died, courageously and with an incredible will. On the way to the hospital, as he was losing consciousness, he said to his parents, "Don't blame yourselves, live!"

Dr. Wilson called me to the emergency room to tell me Kurt had died. I saw his parents and sister sitting together and went to them. We all felt a tremendous loss. He was gone, but the things he had told us would remain forever. Kurt was someone whose whole emotional being changed through the process of having to deal with a life-threatening illness. His method of coping remained the same, the need for concreteness and control, but by opening himself up he enriched the lives of all of us.

Monday morning I woke up to the sound of Carole King singing, ". . . and when the morning sun comes shining through my window, it's good to be alive." It was 6:00 A.M. and I didn't feel very alive. I hustled out of bed and threw on my swimsuit because I knew Kate and Liz would be honking their horn any minute for our lap swim at the local pool. We were crazy, getting up at 6:00 in the pitch black just to get some exercise to improve our bodies! A glass of orange juice and the morning paper sounded much more inviting and sensible!

It was early fall, and as I swam I thought about the few months I had left until I began my time off. In some ways, knowing that I was leaving had made the last weeks easier. I found myself getting less involved with the new patients, knowing I would not be around to see them the next couple of years. It made no sense to build a rapport and develop a support system for them if I was going to leave and withdraw it. Consequently, I directed most of my energy toward the children I had known and worked with over the last three-and-a-half years. Many of them were no longer doing well. Dying at home was becoming a more acceptable alternative to hospitalization, and our doctors were willing to spend the time required if families chose this alternative, including house calls.

The children who were seriously ill had usually been in the hospital for treatments over and over and hated being there. If the parents were comfortable with the idea, we encouraged them to keep their child at home as much as possible. At times it was physically or emotionally impossible, and no one was ever made to feel guilty if they couldn't handle it.

Stephanie, a thirteen-year-old girl with osteogenic sarcoma, was an example of a patient for whom being at home worked well. It was definitely an emotional drain on her family, but she died where she wanted to be—home with her family.

Stephanie was mature beyond her years. She had the ability to give and be concerned about others in the midst of all her own problems. She came to Children's six months after having her leg amputated at her local hospital. Stephanie had been on a chemotherapy drug called high-dose methotrexate. She would be hospitalized and receive the drug for eight weeks, four times a week. It was aggressive therapy but hers was an aggressive disease. Her hair fell out, she was nauseated, and got mouth ulcers, but she continued to fight and take the medication. The tumors continued to grow, or stayed the same. Her attitude was, "I'm doing my part, now you do your part and make these tumors shrink."

She was a feisty young girl with a sense of humor. She had become good friends with many of the other patients and was always offering doctors her advice. Another patient down the hall had the same disease as Stephanie did, equally as serious, with tumors in her lungs, but was extremely depressed. One day Stephanie pulled the doctor aside and said, "You know, you need to make Nancy mad; she needs to get mad." She was right.

Stephanie went home after her eight weeks of treatment. The tumors were stable but not gone. She felt good and was anxious to be with her family. A short while later she suffered a stroke when the disease spread to her brain. Her remaining leg was paralyzed along with her left arm. The doctors talked about more treatments, drugs, surgery, radiation. Stephanie answered the question for them.

She wanted to stay home and she didn't want anything but painkillers. Her parents did not dispute her decision. Off of treatments, Stephanie lived one month. Her mother learned to give her pain shots every two to four hours around the clock, but it wasn't easy. Pain control was difficult to achieve, and when Stephanie would ask for another shot and it wasn't time, it was heartbreaking to watch her suffer. Her father, who loved her dearly, could not go into her bedroom to be with her toward the end. It was too painful for him. Her parents, family, friends, and neighbors all felt helpless, frightened, and exhausted, but they provided the thing most important to her—themselves and home. For them, home care worked.

I had become close to Stephanie during the months I'd known her, but she lived three hours away from the hospital, which made it difficult for me to see her. During her hospitalizations, she had talked about dying, how she wasn't afraid, but had no intention of giving up. She would ask me in the hall or clinic, "How is Rose doing? How is Gary doing? Did he get to go home?" More often than not, those teenagers had died, and I would be the one to have to relay the information to her. I hated that job. Stephanie's response one day was, "You know, Patti, I'm gonna start calling you the bad-news lady. Besides, they all gave up and I'm not giving up."

I called Stephanie on the phone one day during her last month of life, and she said, "I need to talk to you."

I said, "I know." I made arrangements to be out of the hospital the next day.

When I entered her bedroom the first thing she said to me was, "This is a real bummer, isn't it?"

"Yes, Steph, it sure is."

We talked that afternoon about a lot of things. Stephanie wanted me to help her make a will.

"You know, Patti, I have a lot of valuable things."

She asked me what I thought heaven would be like, and I told her my theory. She talked about how much she was going to miss watching her niece and nephew grow up.

"This isn't the way I want it, Patti, but I guess God has other plans. Do you think you could get a minister to come and see me?"

I told her I would. We talked a while longer and held each other's hand. Once again Stephanie asked about some of the other kids, Kurt in particular, since she knew him well. I answered that he was doing okay and had been asking about her too. He died five months later.

When I left that afternoon, I knew I would never see Stephanie again. I would continue to talk with her on the telephone, but we would never again have crutch races in the hall or laugh about Dr. Bleyer's funny ties. She had been a part of my life for nine months, and I felt as if I'd known her forever. Driving home I thought to myself that I wished everyone could know a Stephanie Bailey during their life. A few days before she died at home, Kurt went to see her and they talked as only those two would. She asked her family for a puppy. Ten days before Kurt died he also asked for a puppy. I believe they conspired to make it a little less lonely for their families without them.

Stephanie went into a coma and died peacefully a week

after I had been to visit. She was one tough little girl, thirteen going on seventy.

Many chemotherapy medicines do not require a person to be admitted to the hospital and can be administered on an outpatient basis. One morning as I headed to my office, I stopped in the blood lab to say hi to Allison, a five-year-old who had been coming to the Hematology Clinic as an outpatient for the last three years and had never been admitted to the hospital or experienced any complications from her disease. Her mother was sitting on a chair with Allison on her lap as the lab technician drew a blood sample from Allison's finger. She let out a loud *ouch* and then proceeded to ask for a Snoopy Band-Aid. I asked her how she liked kindergarten, and heard all about Miss Kathleen, her teacher, and her new friend Betsy. Allison's mom told me Allison had only two months of chemotherapy left. It was wonderful to hear that. I thought to myself that I needed to start spending more time in outpatient clinics.

Along with children on treatment, there were also those in the clinic who were finished with their treatments and were seen only for periodic checkups. Those were the kids who were growing into healthy young adults. It was always a joy to sit in the clinic and talk with the fifteen-year-olds whose leukemia had been diagnosed at the age of three or four.

A parent once asked me, "Are you cured of cancer?"

It startled me for a moment, because I thought of myself that way, but never said it out loud. It was almost like if I said it I would jinx myself. The word "cure" had such a sense of finality about it. I felt cured, prayed and hoped I was cured, and lived my life as if I were cured, but who really ever knew? It was always difficult when a parent asked about a child, or a child asked a doctor, "Am I cured?" In childhood cancer, not enough children had survived long enough to be able to give that answer. With

133

more effective drugs and treatments, children are now surviving, unlike fifteen or twenty years ago, and these are the children who will answer the question.

Winter and Christmas were rapidly approaching and I decided I had better tell Dr. Chard and Dr. Hartman of my plans to leave. I found it hard to bring myself to say the words. In my heart I knew I wanted some time off to pursue other interests. They were two fine men who, on all my previous adventures, never said a negative word, only to go, have a good time, and send postcards. I knew I couldn't put it off any longer because many of my friends at the hospital knew I was leaving and I didn't want the doctors to find out through the grapevine.

I went to see Dr. Chard. His response was favorable, but he asked if I would think about taking a six-month-to-one-year leave of absence instead of quitting. It would have to be approved by the hospital administration, but I would have his support. They would leave my position open while I was gone. I was excited at the prospect of being able to take a year off to do anything I wanted and then come back. Both of us knew there was a possibility I wouldn't return, but they were willing to take that chance.

I had made plans to go to Europe and spend time in the British Isles. I wanted to explore the outback of Australia and look into working in a foreign country for a while. Skiing in Idaho and Colorado was high on my priority list for the early months of the winter. As I told Dr. Chard, "I'll be back when my money runs out—could be three months, could be a year."

The group was taking bets! Some thought I would never return once I went away. Laurie thought I'd end up living in a ski resort, skiing winters and golfing summers. The chaplain's bet was a sheep ranch in the outback of Australia. I didn't know. I just wanted a year of exploring and living.

NINETEEN

I HAD ONLY A MONTH TILL I LEFT BUT I DECIDED I needed to get away for a weekend because I was not coping well and needed to forget one of our patients, Teresa Scribner. She was all consumingly on my mind, and my heart ached at the mention of her name. I could no longer be removed, be professional, be objective, or be optimistic. I was angry at God, angry at the limits of medicine, and hated the thing called cancer! *Why are there so many unanswered questions?*

I met Teresa when she was first diagnosed as having Ewing's sarcoma at the age of sixteen. Ewing's sarcoma, a type of bone cancer, is very sensitive to radiation treatments and chemotherapy drugs, so the limb does not need to be amputated. Teresa was a bright, vivacious, typical teenager full of life and energy. She hated the treatments, but she took them for two years, her sixteenth and seventeenth years of life. As time progressed, Teresa felt great, and the medicine was worse than the disease. Several times, she threatened to quit. "I am fine, the tumor is all gone, and these drugs are misery—please, can I stop?"

The answer was No! Dr. Tom Pendergrass told her, "Teresa, there is no sign of your disease, but the treatments

135

are given to make sure all the tumor cells are dead. Hang in there; you're gonna make it."

We fought the battle together. Tom shot in the medicine and I gave pep talks. Teresa cried, then she laughed. "Well you two are a real team. I haven't got a chance of quitting these drugs!"

"Nope, Teresa, we'll come and get you and drag you in here if we have to!"

Teresa and I would go to the cafeteria for a Coke. We'd sit and talk, laugh, and confide in one another. We debated which of the doctors were cutest. She gave Dr. Pendergrass a "10," forgiving him for sticking her five times before he got the needle in her vein.

The end of the two years had finally come. No sign of any recurrent disease and the next chemotherapy shot would be her last one—forever!

Teresa gave me a picture taken of us together and on the back was written:

> Patti, thank you for all your help.
> You've helped me make it through the last two years.
> You did it and—look at me—I did it too!!
> Keep helping everyone like you did me.
>   Love, Your friend, Teresa

I heard my name paged for extension 5241—who was calling me from X-ray?

"Patti, this is Tom, can you come up to X-ray?"

"Sure, Tom, but why?"

"I'll tell you when you get here."

I left what I was doing and went to the elevator. I saw Teresa in the hall.

"Why are you still here? Didn't you get your last shot yet?"

"No, I'm supposed to meet Dr. Pendergrass in the clinic in fifteen minutes. He wanted to look at my final X-rays and then give me my medicine."

"I'll see you in fifteen minutes then," I said. "I wouldn't miss this last injection for anything. Besides, we need to hassle Dr. Pendergrass one final time. You've been too cooperative lately!" I said good-bye and headed for X-ray.

Tom was waiting for me, and in his hand were Teresa's X-rays.

"Patti, these film show tumors in her lungs."

He began to swear and tears welled up in his eyes. I felt tears on my cheeks. *Damn! Why, why, why???*

"How are we going to tell her?"

We put an arm around each other, and I made a mental note to quit for good. I couldn't handle it anymore. We knew there was no easy way. We went downstairs to the clinic, and Tom told Teresa and her mother of his findings. We all cried—there were no words of comfort, no words of wisdom, only a deep sadness. Teresa was scheduled for lung surgery the following week. More chemotherapy was mentioned but no one heard—and no one cared.

I didn't want to see any more patients that day. I felt sick and bewildered. For two years Tom and I had been saying, "Come on Teresa, it's going to be worth it!" I went home that evening and proceeded to drink a fifth of bourbon with a friend. I remembered a quote from a poster I had seen. "Just when you think you've got all the answers, they change the questions." How true it was.

Teresa came into the hospital for lung surgery the following week. We talked. She was scared, but hopeful. I sat with her parents during the surgery, trying to be helpful. Inside I was coming unglued. How much longer until they are done? I thought. Dr. Pendergrass came into the waiting room to talk with us. Surgery was finished and the results were not good. The surgeon found more tumors than showed up on the X-rays and most of them were inoperable. We would have to rely on strong chemotherapy drugs to kill them. I comforted Teresa's parents and two brothers. As always, words seemed so inadequate.

Teresa was told the news and a few days later began the

new chemotherapy drug. It made her sick to her stomach, and she swore as Tom injected the medicine.

"I don't know why I'm even taking this. It didn't work when I did it for two years. Why should it work now?"

We didn't have any answers, only that it might, and that "might" was what her family, Teresa, Dr. Pendergrass, and I were holding on to. After the second treatment, Teresa announced she was not taking any more medicine. The X-rays had shown no change. We argued it took more than two treatments to alter the disease, but she had made up her mind.

"I hate this stuff and I hate myself when I do something I don't believe in. I didn't feel good about me when I took the chemotherapy, and to me that is the most important thing, not if the tumors shrink. I have to feel good about myself."

Teresa made her decision: no more medicine. I couldn't argue, she was right—it was her life and her decision. I could only admire her courage and offer my help and friendship. Teresa went home to die—or live—whichever way you look at it. I believe she went home to live, live the way she believed in living. Her mother shared one of Teresa's poems with me:

> As I approach the end of life
> I pass my hardships, tears, and strife.
> I begin to see and fear the end
> And wish my youth might come again.
> But it never shall for it's not to be
> And I know I'll go when God calls me.
> Hold your tears and tearing hearts
> For I'm happier now, than at the start.

It was Christmas and nearly time to leave Children's. I heard "Jingle Bells" coming from the playroom, and children's laughter echoed in the hall. The doctors were making rounds from room to room, wishing everyone a Merry Christmas. Dr. Pendergrass, with his dark hair and fuzzy beard, squatted to talk to a three-year-old. Dr. Chard, shoulders hunched, walked toward me. We put an arm around each other, and I thought about how far the two of us had come. I thought about the Teresas, Kurts, Lesters, and Kellys I had known and loved those past three years. We had shared together such precious time—time of pain, anger, sadness, death. But there was hope, too, and life. Life! We seldom understood it but we fought for it because we believed in it.

"Patti? Are you getting ready to go home?"

I turned around and found Kevin, a favorite seven-year-old, looking up at me.

"I was thinking about it. Why?"

"Oh, I was just hoping you'd have time for a short game of checkers."

I laughed. "Just a *short* game, huh? Okay, on one condition. I get to be red."

"I have a better idea. We'll race back to my room and the winner will be red. Deal?"

"Deal!" I said. "Dr. Chard, would you be the starter for this great race?"

"Gladly!" he said. "Are you ready?"

"Yes."

"Yes."

"Okay, then. On your mark . . . get set . . . go!"

EPILOGUE

IT IS NOW THE FALL OF 1982, AND ONCE AGAIN I AM looking forward to a birthday—my thirtieth!! I have recently heard several friends complain that they are getting older. But I appreciate how special birthdays really are, gray hairs, flabby thighs, and all. Another year to live. Another year to enjoy.

It doesn't seem as if fifteen years have passed since I was diagnosed as having cancer. I am happy, well, and thriving. Admittedly I am lucky, but thankfully, more and more children and adults today are surviving cancer and leading normal, healthy lives. Although there has been no recurrence of my cancer, I continue to have a chest X-ray and checkup once every two years. I still see Dr. Burgess and he still asks me why I do not wear my leg. He always lets me know when there have been improvements in artificial limbs, so he hasn't given up on me. He still calls me his "miracle girl."

Although I do not wear my artificial leg much at all, I occasionally think about having a new one made and trying again. It has become much easier and quicker through the years to do everything on crutches, but I recall Dr. Burgess's words when I was only seventeen. "It's like skiing, you have to keep practicing over and over until it becomes natural."

Using crutches all the time still means answering people's questions about "what happened?" or "where is your leg?" That has not changed and I am still "talking alligators." My remaining leg is strong and my balance is great. I often balance on my one leg when I take a shower, wash dishes, make beds, or do the hundreds of other things that make up everyday life. At times, rather than using my crutches, I will just hop from one place to another. My little four-year-old neighbor says that I would make a great Easter Bunny. I tend to agree!

I've found—or created—a way to do most everything I've wanted to do, with the exception of jogging. As I watch people jog along looking healthy and sweaty, for a few seconds I feel sorry for myself and wish I could participate, but then I chuckle to myself and realize that even if I had two legs, I probably wouldn't enjoy running. Disciplining myself to swim three times a week is hard enough!

There are times, however, when I do get frustrated. Times when I wish I could just get up and walk without reaching for a pair of crutches. Times when I'd like to go for a bike ride or swim and not have people stare at me or tell me how amazing I am. Times when I'd just like to be like everyone else. I was recently walking through a park with my boyfriend when I overheard a little boy say to his father, "Look at that girl. She broke her leg and forgot the cast." I had to smile and felt complimented that he considered me a "girl" and not a lady!

After leaving Children's Hospital in 1979 I enjoyed traveling around the world for a year. When I returned to Seattle I again worked at the hospital until my position was cut because of lack of funding. Nobody denied the importance of my job and the benefits to the children and their families, but the reality remained that the funding was not available for my programs and position.

I then decided that a complete career change might be good for me so I went into medical sales, using my occupational-therapy skills selling home health equipment. I have enjoyed it, and the business world has taught me a great deal.

I continue to run a monthly children's group on a volunteer basis and get much more from working with these kids than I am ever able to give them. I will never forget the group's first meeting two years ago. There were ten kids, all in different stages of their disease. We had made pizza for dinner and were sitting in a circle talking about how they coped with getting so many "needle pokes" all the time. After our discussion the kids decided they would like to elect officers and make the group into a special club. I thought it sounded like a great idea, so nominations were opened. They proceeded to nominate each other and elected a president, a secretary, and a treasurer. Suddenly eight-year-old Darrin looked very serious.

"We forgot to elect a vice-president."

Another group member said, "What do we need a vice-president for?"

Darrin quickly replied, "In case the president dies of cancer, stupid!"

I was caught off guard for a moment, but then another child agreed, and soon we had elected a vice-president. So began my job as leader of this group which not only has many thoughts and feelings about having cancer, but also many ideas about living.

Some of you may be wondering what happened to Crazy George. Well, he is still "crazy," and we continue to get together during the winter and keep in touch by telephone the rest of the year. He is still "flying" down mountains as well as jumping out of planes. He recently acquired a hot-air balloon, and I have lived to tell the tale of my first ride with him.

Lots of changes have taken place through the years, and

this thirtieth year will be no different. Although I am still single, that too may change in the near future. I continue to look for new challenges and adventures, and I've never been happier or more ready to get on with my life.